Ovarian Cancer in Elderly Patients

Gilles Freyer

Editor

Ovarian Cancer in Elderly Patients

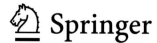 Springer

Editor
Gilles Freyer
HCL Cancer Institute
Medical Oncology, and Université de Lyon
Lyon
France

ISBN 978-3-319-23587-5   ISBN 978-3-319-23588-2   (eBook)
DOI 10.1007/978-3-319-23588-2

Library of Congress Control Number: 2015954241

Springer Cham Heidelberg New York Dordrecht London

Printed on acid-free paper

Springer International Publishing AG Switzerland is part of Springer Science+Business Media
(www.springer.com)

Preface

This practical book provides up-to-date information on the particular features of ovarian cancer in older women and the best management approach. Various relevant topics are covered. Guidance is provided on geriatric assessment, pathology, molecular biology, diagnosis, and treatment. The various treatment options are carefully explained, covering surgical approaches, chemotherapy as a first-line strategy, use of anti-angiogenic agents, and treatment of relapse. The cognitive problems that may arise in elderly women during and after treatment of ovarian cancer are documented, with advice on response. Guidance is also provided on the design of clinical trials, and current directions in biological research are reviewed. This book will be of value to both practitioners and researchers with an interest in ovarian cancer and the elderly.

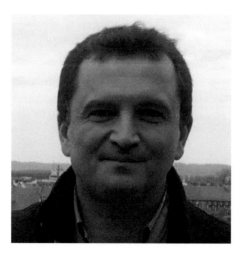

Lyon, France   Gilles Freyer, MD, PhD

Contents

Systemic Treatment of Cancer in the Older-Aged Person

Lodovico Balducci

Contents

In the older patient, the benefits of systemic cancer treatment may be lessened due to decreased life expectancy and the risk of complications may be augmented due to diminished functional reserve [1, 2]. In all cases, the cost of cancer care increases with age due to prevention and management of adverse events [3].

This chapter explores ways to deliver value in cancer care to older individuals, that is, to obtain the best outcome with the lowest risk of complications and at the lowest cost [4, 5].

Definition and Assessment of Physiologic Age

Aging [6, 7] involves a progressive restriction in the functional reserve of multiple organ systems that is intertwined with increased prevalence of chronic conditions (polymorbidity) including the so-called geriatric syndromes and with declining resources and social support. While not unique of aging, geriatric syndromes become more common with advanced age [8]. They include dementia, depression,

L. Balducci, MD
Moffitt Cancer Center, 12902 Magnolia Dr, Tampa, FL, 33612, USA
e-mail: Lodovico.balducci@moffitt.org

© Springer International Publishing Switzerland 2016
G. Freyer (ed.), *Ovarian Cancer in Elderly Patients*,
DOI 10.1007/978-3-319-23588-2_1

incontinence, falls, spontaneous fractures, dizziness, neglect and abuse, and failure to thrive and they compromise the ability of a person to live independently.

A number of physiologic changes occurring with age may be comprehended in the term "allostasis" that means loss of ability to recover the original physiologic equilibrium after stress [9]. The best known form of allostasis in the elderly is chronic inflammation [10], which is associated with most manifestations of aging, including geriatric syndromes, polymorbidity, sarcopenia, immune suppression, and functional dependence. Like inflammation, endocrine senescence may cause a catabolic status in the older persons, with increased insulin resistance, increased circulating levels of adrenal corticoid, and a diminished production of sexual hormones.

At a cellular level, aging is characterized by a progressive loss of the ability of cellular self-renewal [11, 12]. This is due in part to a progressive telomere shortening [9] and in part to development of genomic alterations that trigger the activity of antiproliferative genes. Among these, the gatekeeper P16INK4a has been studied in several experimental aging models as well as in clinical situations [13].

Aging is universal but it occurs at a different rate in different individuals. It is poorly reflected in chronologic age and medical decisions in older individuals should rather be based on physiologic age [6]. In the case of cancer treatment, the questions facing the practitioner include:

Is the patient going to die of cancer or with cancer?
Is the patient going to live long enough to suffer the complications of cancer?
Is the patient able to tolerate the treatment of cancer?

In addition to these questions, one may ask whether cancer treatment may lead to worsening disability in cancer survivors [14]. Loss of independence is the worst threat to the quality of life of an older individual so much so that prolongation of active life expectancy is considered a major goal of medical treatment [14].

Several laboratory tests have been proposed to estimate the physiologic age of older individuals. The inflammatory index is calculated as the log of interleukin 6+2logs of the concentration of tumor necrosis factor receptor 1(TNFR1) in the circulation and has been validated for predicting the risk of mortality at 10 years in two cohorts of several thousand individuals aged 65 and over [10]. However, it is not validated in individuals with chronic diseases and in particular with cancer. The length of leukocyte telomere is inadequate to compare the age of different individuals given the high degree of interindividual variability [15]. The determination of the P16INK4a is promising but requires the sampling of normal tissues [16]. Also, this test has not been validated for estimating the survival and functional reserve of older individuals.

Currently, a comprehensive geriatric assessment (CGA) (Table 1.1) [17] is considered the most useful instrument to estimate the risk of cancer-unrelated mortality [18] and to predict the risk of chemotherapy-related toxicity in older cancer patients [19, 20]. In addition, the CGA allows to uncover conditions that may compromise the treatment of cancer, including comorbidity, malnutrition, and inadequate social

Table 1.1 Examples of CGA and potential clinical applications

7	Relation to life expectancy, functional dependence, and tolerance to stress
	Relation to life expectancy and tolerance to stress
	Relation to life expectancy and dependence
	Relation to survival; may indicate motivation to receive treatment
	Reversible condition; possible relationship to survival
	Risk of drug interactions
	Relationship to survival Functional dependence

support. For these reasons, the guidelines of the National Cancer Center Network recommend that some form of CGA be performed in all individuals aged 70+ [17].

It is important to avoid possible misinterpretation of the CGA. First of all, it should not be applied to acute situations. To diagnose functional dependence, the inability to perform ADLs or IADLs should be present as a chronic condition, not just during an acute episode that compels the patient to be bedridden. The same should be said of the so-called geriatric syndromes. Delirium is a geriatric syndrome if it occurs in the presence of a mild upper respiratory or urinary infection or upon administration of drugs that do not cause delirium commonly. Falls are a geriatric syndrome if they are frequent and without apparent causes. Second, a person who is able to compensate for a disability should not be considered dependent in ADLs (e.g., a paraplegic who is able to use a wheelchair is not dependent in transferring).

Dependence in ADLs, the presence of one or more geriatric syndromes, and severe comorbid conditions generally purport a very limited life expectancy and treatment tolerance and the majority of these individuals may be suitable only for palliative care. In any case, each situation should be evaluated individually and treated accordingly.

Figure 1.1 illustrates the approach recommended to the treatment of older individuals, based on the CGA. Alternative treatments may include chemotherapy at lower doses or alternative forms of chemotherapy that may be effective, albeit not as effective as the standard treatment. It may also include management of reversible conditions that prevent the administration of the most effective therapy (such as malnutrition or inadequate caregiver).

Ultimately, the treatment-related decision will be negotiated with the patient and his/her caregiver. The CGA allows the practitioner to provide objective information related to the potential benefits and risks of the treatment, to foster realistic expectations, and to facilitate an informed decision. In a randomized study of patients with metastatic non-small cell lung cancer, this approach has led to the best quality care of these patients, that is, to a more prolonged survival at a decreased cost and with improved patient satisfaction [21]. These results were obtained because full information led to earlier participation in clinical trials, reduced use of third-line chemotherapy and of the intensive care, and better planning for end-of-life care.

Clearly, the management of the older cancer patient with systemic treatment is a team endeavor that involves the cooperation of aging and cancer specialists. While

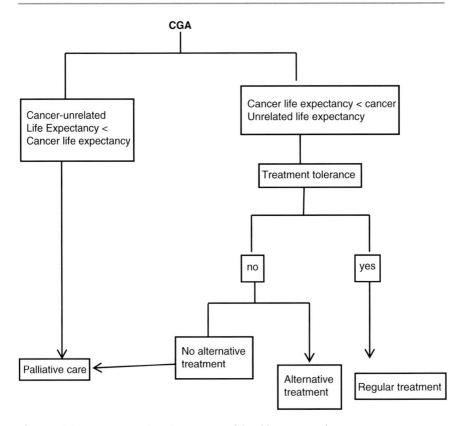

Fig. 1.1 CGA based approach to the treatment of the older cancer patient

it may appear time and cost intensive, the team approach may eventually prevent the wasting of limited health-care resources, by avoiding futile treatment and its potential complications.

Controversy lingers concerning the best form of CGA and as to whether a full-fledged CGA is necessary in all patients. A number of investigators reported that time-sparing screening instruments, including the vulnerable elderly survey-13 (VES-13) [22], the study of osteoporotic fractures test (SOF) [23], the Groningen index [24], and the G-test [25], are as sensitive as a full CGA for the detection of aging-related abnormalities, while other authors did not confirm these findings [26, 27]. At the very minimum, it is important to assess those elements necessary to predict mortality and chemotherapy-related toxicity including ADLs, IADLs, polymorbidity, and nutritional and cognitive status [18–20]. Whenever the time allows it, the investigation of all domains of the CGA appears desirable.

Pharmacology of Aging

Aging may be associated with a number of pharmacologic changes described in Table 1.2 [28].

Table 1.2 Pharmacologic changes of aging

Pharmacokinetics
  Absorption
  Volume of distribution
  Metabolism
  Renal excretion
  Hepatic excretion
	The effects of aging on absorption are unknown. It is reasonable to assume a progressive decrease in absorption due to atrophic gastritis, decreased gastric motility, and decreased splanchnic circulation
	Changes in body composition with increased fat and decreased water content
	Hepatic metabolism is reduced from progressive loss of liver mass and decreased splanchnic circulation
	Glomerular filtration rate declines with age in virtually all individuals
	Biliary excretion seems to remain intact

Pharmacodynamics
  Hematopoietic system
  Mucosa epithelium
  Heart
  Peripheral nervous system
  Central nervous system
	Decreased concentration of early hematopoietic progenitors, decreased lymphocytic production; homing abnormality that may reduce the concentration of early progenitors in the marrow
	Decreased epithelial stem cells and increased proliferation of differentiated cells
	Reduction in myocardial sarcomeres; increased fibrosis and degenerative processes (amyloid)
	Increased degenerative processes
	Atrophy and increase in degenerative processes with decreased circulation

Pharmacokinetics Data on drug absorption are wanted. This information is critical, given the rapid development of new oral antineoplastic agents during the past two decades. Data limited to imatinib [29] and oral idarubicin [30] suggest that the absorption of oral agents is unaffected by age. These studies included only elderly in good general conditions and under 85. It is reasonable to expect that bioavailability of an oral drug may decrease in some older individuals due to a combination of factors that include reduced splanchnic circulation, decreased gastrointestinal secretions, and mucosal atrophy [28]. Another issue related to oral drug is adherence to the treatment plans, as many older individuals are taking multiple medications and may find it difficult to remember to take each medication at the appointed time. An additional difficulty includes the presence of swallowing disorders, whose prevalence increases with age.

The decreased body total water content is associated with decreased volume of distribution and increased levels of water-soluble drugs in the circulation that may purport increased toxicity. The volume of distribution of hydrosoluble agents may also be determined in part by the concentration of plasmatic proteins and of hemoglobin, to which these drugs may be bound [31].

Renal excretion and hepatic metabolism of drugs are universally decreased with age. While the decline in glomerular filtration rate may be easily accounted for by calculating the creatinine clearance, a clinical test of hepatic metabolism is still wanted.

Pharmacodynamics As already mentioned, a number of age-related changes in target organs may be associated with increased hematopoietic, mucosal, cardiac, and neurological toxicity. The risk of chemotherapy-induced neutropenia, of neutropenic infections, and of lethal neutropenic infections increases with the age of the patients [32]. Data on the incidence of chemotherapy-induced anemia and thrombo-cytopenia in older individuals are wanted, but it is clear that the prevalence of ane-mia and the risk of anemia-related medical complications increase with the age of the patients [31]. In about 50 % of cases, anemia in older individuals is reversible and should be aggressively managed with the double goal to improve the patient's quality of life and energy levels and to prevent chemotherapy-related complications that are more frequent in the presence of anemia.

Mucositis, especially when it is associated to diarrhea and with dysphagia, may represent a cause of rapid fluid depletion and should be administered very aggressively.

Peripheral neuropathy is a common complication of platinum derivatives, alka-loids, and epothilones and it may be disabling for older individuals.

Cardiotoxicity is a complication of treatment with anthracyclines and anthra-cenediones and of the monoclonal antibody trastuzumab [33]. The risk of this com-plication increases with age. The cardiotoxicity from trastuzumab is reversible in the majority of cases upon drug withdrawal.

The information related to the toxicity of new targeted agents in older individuals is limited [34]. In general, these agents are better tolerated than cytotoxic chemo-therapy, but even for them, the risk of complications seems to increase with age. In addition to the cardiotoxicity of trastuzumab [33] already mentioned, the risk of hypertension and bleeding with bevacizumab, of severe dermatitis with tyrosine kinase inhibitors (TKI) and anti-EGFR antibodies, and of fluid retention with ima-tinib is of special concern. In most cases, it is not clear whether the increased risk of toxicity is due to altered pharmacokinetics or pharmacodynamics (increased sus-ceptibility of target tissues to treatment complications). In the case of imatinib, this issue has been studied in details and the increased toxicity was associated with an increased AUC of the drug in older individuals.

Late Complications of Cancer Treatment Cancer chemotherapy may accelerate the aging process [35]. Almost 40 % of individuals treated for cancer during their child-hood develop signs of frailty in their 30s versus 10 % of non-cancer controls. In 33 adult women with early-stage breast cancer [36], adjuvant chemotherapy has been associated with increased expression of aging markers (p16(INK4a) and ARF) in the tissues and increased concentration of inflammatory cytokines in the blood and these changes persisted for at least 1 year. These findings suggest that cytotoxic chemotherapy may accelerate the development of functional dependence in older individuals.

Age is a risk factor for chemotherapy-induced acute myelogenous leukemia and myelodysplasia [37] and for cardiovascular dysfunction [37].

It is not clear whether the incidence of dementia increases in older patients treated with chemotherapy. What is clear is that the risk of cognitive dysfunctions increases and cognitive dysfunctions are a major cause of concern and of deteriora-tion of quality of life [14].

Fatigue is the most common chronic complication of cancer chemotherapy [14], and fatigue in the elderly is associated both with functional dependence and increased mortality [38].

Osteoporosis is a major complication of hormonal treatment of cancer and in particular of aromatase inhibitors in the management of breast cancer and of androgen deprivation in the management of prostate cancer [39].

Conclusions

Older cancer patients may benefit from the systemic treatment of cancer to the same extent as younger individuals. However, the risk of treatment-related toxicity may be increased due to reduced functional reserve. The NCCN committee on aging has issued some guidelines for the management of cancer in older patients with chemotherapy [17]. These include:

- Some form of CGA as part of the initial evaluation of individuals 70 and older. The CGA may provide information related to the risk of cancer-unrelated mortality, the risk of chemotherapy-related toxicity, and the presence of conditions that may preclude the safe administration of chemotherapy.
- Adjustment of the initial dose of chemotherapy to the glomerular filtration rate. Subsequent doses may be escalated or de-escalated according to the presence or absence of complications.
- Prophylactic use of filgrastim and pegfilgrastim in patients 65 and older for chemotherapy regimens of dose intensity comparable to CHOP.

In addition to these, it is reasonable to recommend aggressive prevention of fatigue with daily exercise and adequate nutrition intake [14] and prevention of bone loss from hormonal treatment. This may include regular intake of calcium and vitamin D and use of bisphosphonates [38].

References

1. Balducci L, Aapro M. Complicated and complex: helping the older cancer patient to exit the labyrinth. J Ger Oncol. 2014;5:116–8.
2. Brighi N, Balducci L, Biasco G. Cancer in the elderly: is it time for palliative care in geriatric oncology? J Ger Oncol. 2014;5:197–203.
3. Yabroff KL, Lamont EB, Marotto A, et al. Cost of care for elderly cancer patients in the United States. J Natl Cancer Inst. 2008;100:630–41.
4. Ganz PA. Institute of medicine report on delivery of high quality cancer care. J Oncol Pract. 2014;10:193–5.
5. Curtman GD, Morissey S, Drazen SM. High value health care: a sustainable proposition. N Engl J Med. 2013;369:1163–4.
6. Balducci L. Frailty: a common pathway in aging and cancer. Interdisc Top Gerontol. 2013;38:61–72.
7. Popa MA, Wallace KJ, Brunello A, et al. Potential drug interactions and chemotoxicity in older patients with cancer receiving chemotherapy. J Ger Oncol. 2014, pii: S1879-4068(14)00065-4. doi:10.1016/j.jgo.2014.04.002.
8. Mcrae PJ, Peele NM, Walker PJ, et al. Geriatric Syndromes in individuals admitted to vascular and urology surgical units. J Am Ger Soc. 2014. doi:10.1111/jgs.12827.
9. Zalli A, Carvalho LA, Lin J, et al. Shorter telomeres with higher telomerase activity are associated with raised allostatic load and impoverished social resources. Proc Natl Acad Sci. 2014;111:4519–24.

10. Varadhan R, Yao W, Matteini A, et al. Simple biologically informed inflammatory index of 2 serum cytokines predicts 10 year all cause mortality in older adults. J Gerontol A Biol Sci Med Sci. 2014;69:165–73.
11. Rodler F, Campisi J. Four faces of cellular senescence. J Cell Biol. 2011;142:547–56.
12. Berman AE, Leontleva OV, Natarajan V, et al. Recent progress in genetics of aging: senescence and longevity focusing on cancer-related genes. Oncotarget. 2012;3:1522–32.
13. Chandler H, Peters G. Stressing the cell cycle in senescence and aging. Curr Opin Cell Biol. 2013;25:765–71.
14. Balducci L, Fossa LD. Rehabilitation of older cancer patients. Acta Oncol. 2013;52:233–8.
15. Bendix L, Thinggaard M, Fenger M, et al. Longitudinal changes of leukocyte telomere length and mortality in humans. J Gerontol A Biol Sci Med Sci. 2014;69:231–9.
16. Choudhery MS, Badowski M, Muise A, et al. Donor age negatively impacts adipose tissue derived mesenchymal stem cell expansion and differentiation. J Transl Med. 2014;12:8. doi:10.1186/1479-5876-12-8.
17. Hurria A, Wildes T, Blair ST, et al. Senior Adult Oncology> version 2 2014. J Natl Compr Cancer Ntw. 2014;12:82–126.
18. Yourman LG, Lee SJ, Schonberg MA, et al. Prognostic indices for older adults: a systematic review. JAMA. 2012;307:182–92.
19. Extermann M, Boler I, Reich RR, et al. Predicting the risk of chemotherapy toxicity in older patients: the Chemotherapy Risk Assessment Scale in High Age Patients (CRASH) score. Cancer. 2012;118:3377–86.
20. Hurria A, Togawa K, Mohile ST, et al. Predicting chemotherapy toxicity in older adults with cancer. A prospective multicenter study. J Clin Oncol. 2011;29:3457–65.
21. Yoong J, Park ER, Greer AJ, et al. Early palliative care in assessment lung cancer qualitative study. JAMA. 2013;173:283–90.
22. Luciani A, Ascione B, Bertuzzi C, et al. Detecting disability in older patients with cáncer: comparison between comprehensive geriatric assessment and vulnerable elderly survey. J Clin Oncol. 2010;28:2046–50.
23. Luciani A, Dottorini L, Battisti N. Screening elderly cancer patients for disability: comparison of study of osteoporotic fracture index and comprehensive geriatric assessment (CGA). Ann Oncol. 2013;24:469–74.
24. Baitar A, von Fraevenhove F, Vanderbroek A, et al. Evaluation of the groningen frailty indicator and the G8 questionnaire as screening tools for frailty in older patients with cancer. J Ger Oncol. 2013;4:32–8.
25. Bellera CA, Rainfray M, Mathoulin-Pelissier S, et al. Screening older cancer patients: first evaluation of the G8 geriatric screening tool. Ann Oncol. 2012;23:2166–72.
26. Smets IH, Kempen GI, Janssen-Heijnen ML, et al. Four screening instruments for frailty in older patients with and without cancer: a diagnostic study. BMC Geriatr. 2014;14:26. doi:10.1186/1471-2318-14-26.
27. Biganzoli L, Boni L, Becheri D, et al. Evaluation of the cardiovascular health study instrument and of the Vulnerable Elderly Survey 13 (VES-13) in elderly cancer patients. Are we still missing the right screening tool? Ann Oncol. 2013;24:494–500.
28. Hoffe S, Balducci L. Cancer and aging: general considerations. Clin Geriatr Med. 2012;28:1–12.
29. Latagliata R, Ferrero D, Iurlo A, et al. Imatinib in very elderly patients with chronic myeloid leukemia in chronic stage: a retrospective study. Drugs Aging. 2013;30:629–37.
30. Crivellari D, Lombardi D, Spazzapan S, et al. New oral drugs in older patients: a review of idarubicin in elderly patients. Crit Rev Oncol Hematol. 2004;49:153–63.
31. Balducci L. Anemia, fatigue and aging. Transfus Clin Biol. 2010;17:375–81.
32. Crawford J, Armitage J, Balducci L, et al. Myeloid growth factors. J Natl Compr Cancer Netw. 2013;11:1266–90.
33. Tsai HT, Isaacs C, Fu AZ. Risk of cardiovascular events from trastuzumab in elderly persons with breast cancer: a population based study. Breast Cancer Res Treat. 2014;144:163–70.

34. Gonsalves W, Ganti AK. Targeted anticancer therapy in the elderly. Crit Rev Oncol Hematol. 2011;78:227–42.
35. Henderson TO, Ness KK, Cohen HJ. Accelerated aging in cancer survivors: from pediatrics to geriatrics. Am Soc Clin Oncol Ed Book. 2014;34:e423–30.
36. Sanoff HK, Deal AM, Krishnamurthy J, et al. Effects of cytotoxic chemotherapy on markers of cellular age in patients with breast cancer. J Natl Cancer Inst. 2014;106(4):dju057. doi:10.1093/jnci/dju05.
37. Petrelli F, Borgonovo K, Cabiddu M, et al. Mortality, leukemic risk and cardiovascular toxicity of adjuvant anthracycline and taxane chemotherapy in breast cancer: a meta-analysis. Breast Cancer Res Treat. 2012;135:335–46.
38. Moreh E, Jacobs JM, Stessman J. Fatigue, function, and mortality in older adults. J Gerontol Biol Sci Med Sci. 2010;65:887–95.
39. Balducci L. Bone complications of cancer treatment in the elderly. Oncology. 2010;24:741–7.

Cognitive Function During and After Treatment in Elderly Ovarian Cancer Patients

2

Marie Lange and Florence Joly

Contents

Beyond the difficulties with attention, concentration, and memory reported by cancer patients, it has become increasingly apparent that cytotoxic drugs given for non-central nervous system tumors might have side effects on cognitive functioning. This phenomenon, called *chemobrain*, has been mainly studied among young breast cancer patients treated with chemotherapy. Besides adding to the other side effects of treatment, these difficulties have a negative impact on quality of life [1]. In

M. Lange
INSERM U1086 "Cancers et préventions", Service de Recherche Clinique, Centre François Baclesse, 3 avenue général Harris, 14076 Caen cedex 05, France
e-mail: m.lange@baclesse.fr

F. Joly (✉)
INSERM U1086 "Cancers et préventions", Service de Recherche Clinique, Centre François Baclesse, CHU de Caen, 3 avenue général Harris, 14076 Caen cedex 05, France
e-mail: f.joly@baclesse.fr

© Springer International Publishing Switzerland 2016
G. Freyer (ed.), *Ovarian Cancer in Elderly Patients*,
DOI 10.1007/978-3-319-23588-2_2

11

comparison to breast cancer patients, there is a paucity of research on the *chemobrain* in ovarian cancer women and none has focused on elderly patients. Nevertheless, patients with ovarian cancer may be at risk of developing cognitive disorders. More than half of patients with ovarian cancer are over 65 at diagnosis [2] and age is a risk factor for ovarian cancer and cognitive impairments. Furthermore, the management of ovarian cancer includes initial extensive surgery with long anesthesia and several courses of chemotherapy that could induce cognitive disorders impacting quality of life [3]. The recent introduction of maintenance therapy with antiangiogenic agents such as bevacizumab is another factor that may have negative effects on the cognitive functions of these patients [4].

Introduction: Concept of *Chemobrain*

The term *chemobrain* refers to impairments of episodic memory, working memory, executive functions, attention, and information processing speed [5, 6], and recent neuroimaging studies have revealed the fronto-subcortical effect of chemotherapy [7, 8]. In practice, patients experience difficulties regarding memory information retrieval and the memorization of information while processing. The impairment also concerns the capacity to adapt behavior to new situations, to concentrate, and to process information quickly. These impairments are assessed by neuropsychological tests.

These objective cognitive dysfunctions have been reported to affect 15–50 % of chemotherapy-treated patients and are usually moderate [9]. Cognitive decline has been observed to persist in subgroups of patients from 1 year [10, 11] to 10–20 years [12, 13] posttreatment (for a review, see [14]). Most of the studies to date have been conducted among breast cancer patients and recent longitudinal studies showed that about 20–30 % of breast cancer patients have cognitive impairment before any adjuvant treatment [15]. This indicates that, besides exposure to cytotoxic drugs, other factors including the biological adverse effects of cancer itself, genetic factors, psychological distress related to the diagnosis, fatigue, and postoperative dysfunctions are involved, suggesting an impact of cancer as a whole on cognitive functions [16, 17].

Many patients complain of cognitive decline even if they perform well on neuropsychological tests, and in most cases, no relationship between subjective complaints and objective cognitive deficits has been found [18, 19]. Similar findings have been made in ovarian cancer patients with some (48 %) reporting a significant decline in perceived cognitive functioning during chemotherapy, although their objective scores were not declined [20]. These frequent complaints (21–90 % of patients with breast cancer [19]) may persist several years after the end of treatment [21] and are commonly associated with anxiety and depression.

This paper presents the state of the art regarding cancer and treatment-induced cognitive impairment in ovarian cancer patients with the focus on elderly patients. The specificities of elderly cancer patients are discussed and the mechanisms explaining the impact of cancer treatments on cognition are presented. Finally, recommendations are made regarding the evaluation of cognitive assessment in older ovarian cancer patients and its practical feasibility.

Cognition and Ovarian Cancer Patients

Despite the multiple courses of chemotherapy included in the normal management of ovarian cancer patients, little is known about cognitive functions of these patients in comparison to other cancer populations such as breast cancer [22].

Although it is well known that 5-FU or methotrexate can induce cognitive decline [23], data are scarce about the impact of carboplatin and paclitaxel, the mainstays of treatment in ovarian cancer. Paclitaxel can cause peripheral nervous system toxicities such as paresthesia, dysesthesia, and muscle weakness. It may have similar effects on the central nervous system that could result in cognitive impairment, as suggested by recent imaging studies [24]. There is also emerging evidence suggesting that vascular endothelial growth factor (VEGF) has a role in brain cognition and that VEGF inhibitors may induce neurotoxic effects on patients' cognitive function [4]. Some clinical case series have been published reporting reversible cognitive disorders such as confusion, memory loss, and word-finding difficulties with sunitinib while bevacizumab reportedly induces posterior encephalopathy syndromes even in normotensive patients [25, 26].

Over the last decade, only four small studies using neuropsychological tests have assessed the impact of ovarian cancer and its treatments on objective cognitive functions. Three of these are longitudinal and the other concerns long-term survivors (Table 2.1).

Mayerhofer et al. [27] assessed cognitive functioning before treatment, after 3 cycles, and at the end of chemotherapy (paclitaxel/carboplatin) in 28 women (median age 63) with advanced ovarian cancer. Attention and motor skills were assessed with neuropsychological tests. Before starting chemotherapy, 82 % of patients presented cognitive impairment (mainly motor skills), and high rates of anxiety were observed. During and after treatment, patients with initial deficits did not deteriorate. On the other hand, a significant improvement on attention scores was found ($p < 0.05$) probably owing to practice effects. Thus, the results showed no signs of neuropsychological worsening after paclitaxel/carboplatin chemotherapy.

Hensley et al. [20] studied the impact of chemotherapy (paclitaxel, gemcitabine, and carboplatin) on cognitive functioning and quality of life in 20 women with advanced ovarian, peritoneal, or fallopian tube cancer (median age 54). Four evaluations were performed: before treatment, after cycles 3 and 6, and 6 months after completion of chemotherapy. Patients had a short objective (2 tests of executive functions and processing speed) and subjective assessment with a self-report questionnaire investigating memory and concentration. Results showed that objective cognitive functioning did not decline during or after chemotherapy. More highly educated women (i.e., more than 16 years of education) reported a decline in their concentration, memory, and emotional well-being during treatment. Cognitive complaints returned to baseline levels 6 months after completion of chemotherapy.

Table 2.1 Cognitive studies in women with ovarian cancer

Study	Patients	Chemotherapy type	Time of assessment	Age	Cognitive assessment	Results
Mayerhofer et al. [27]	Patients with advanced ovarian cancer ($n=28$)	Paclitaxel/carboplatin	Before CT, after cycle 3, and after CT completion	Median: 63 (54–69)	NP tests: attention, motor skills	82 % of patients had impairment before CT (mainly motor skills) No decline during or after CT Improvement in attention scores
Hensley et al. [20]	Patients with advanced ovarian, peritoneal, or fallopian tube cancer ($n=20$)	Paclitaxel, carboplatin, gemcitabine	Before CT, after cycles 3 and 6, and 6 months after CT completion	Median: 54 (25–70)	2 NP tests: executive functions, processing speed, short-term and working memories Subjective assessment	No decline during or after CT
Hess et al. [28]	Patients with advanced ovarian or primary peritoneal cancer ($n=27$)	Platinum-based therapy	Before CT, after cycles 3 and 6	Mean 59 (40–82)	NP computerized tests: attention, processing speed, reaction time Subjective assessment	92 % decline at cycle 3 and 86 % decline at cycle 6 (compared to baseline) About 40 % of patients had ≥2 domains impaired
Correa et al. [29]	Ovarian cancer survivors in complete remission ($n=22$, group 1) vs. ovarian cancer survivors with recurrent disease receiving CT ($n=26$, group 2)	Mainly paclitaxel and carboplatin	Cross-sectional: 5–10 years from diagnosis	Group 1: 62 ± 9.2 Group 2: 60 ± 9.1	Battery of standardized NP tests: attention, executive functions, learning and memory abilities	No difference between patient groups 28 % of patients had cognitive impairment

CT chemotherapy, *HT* hormonal therapy, *NP* neuropsychological

Moreover, depression and overall quality of life scores did not change significantly during or at completion of chemotherapy. However, cognitive assessment was insufficiently detailed in this study so it is difficult to draw any conclusions.

Hess et al. [28] investigated objective and subjective cognitive changes among women with newly diagnosed advanced ovarian cancer ($n=27$, mean age$=59$) with assessments prior to chemotherapy and at the third and sixth cycle of chemotherapy (platinum-based therapy). Objective assessment consisted in web-based evaluation of attention, processing speed, and reaction time. Results showed that 92 % and 86 % of patients demonstrated cognitive declines at least on one domain from baseline to cycle 3 and from baseline to cycle 6, respectively. Forty-eight percent and 41 % of patients had at least two domains impaired at cycle 3 and cycle 6, respectively. Nevertheless, higher levels of memory complaints were reported before than after chemotherapy.

One study focused on the cognitive functioning of long-term survivors of ovarian cancer. The cross-sectional study of Correa et al. [29] in women diagnosed with ovarian cancer 5–10 years prior to study enrollment compared neuropsychological performances of women in complete remission ($n=22$) with that of women who had recurrent disease and were receiving chemotherapy ($n=26$). Patients in both groups received chemotherapy prior to enrollment (mainly paclitaxel and carboplatin). Twenty-eight percent of patients had cognitive impairment, which is greater than would be expected considering healthy population norms ($p=0.03$). In the group of survivors who were treated for a disease relapse, there was a trend for a higher frequency of impairment than that reported in healthy population norms ($p=0.051$), whereas this result was not found in women in complete remission. In the group of recurrent disease, there was a moderate negative correlation between the number of prior chemotherapies and performances on tests of attention and executive functions. Furthermore, no significant difference was found between these two groups of patients on tests of attention, learning and memory abilities, and executive functions or depression.

Cognitive complaints have also been reported in studies using the self-report questionnaire QLQ-C30 of the European Organization for Research and Treatment Cancer (EORTC) in ovarian cancer patients [22]. With this questionnaire, a decline in perceived cognitive function was observed in some but not all studies [22]. However, the QLQ-C30 includes only 2 items dedicated to cognition and it was not designed and developed specifically to assess cognitive complaints.

In summary, longitudinal studies are not consensual regarding the deleterious impact of chemotherapy on cognitive functioning in ovarian cancer patients. These inconsistent findings are likely to be in part related to methodical issues [22]. The studies included small sample sizes and no control group to help to delineate the effect of chemotherapy on cognition (cancer patients not treated by chemotherapy and healthy controls to apprehend practice effects), and only a few neuropsychological tests were used and not all the domains likely to be affected by chemotherapy were assessed. Furthermore, cognitive complaints were not assessed with a specific questionnaire like the Functional Assessment of Cancer Therapy–Cognitive Function (FACT-Cog), which has been validated with cancer patients [30].

Moreover, the longitudinal studies focused only on the acute effect of chemotherapy, and the impact of antiangiogenic agents such as bevacizumab in association with chemotherapy and in maintenance was not assessed.

The four studies presented were not dedicated to elderly patients and only a few older women with ovarian cancer were included.

Additional research with a longitudinal design and following the International Cognition and Cancer Task Force recommendations [31] is therefore needed to apprehend more precisely the contribution of the disease, treatments, and other risk factors on cognitive functioning linked to aging.

Elderly Cancer Patients

The *chemobrain* has been particularly studied among women treated for breast cancer, mainly in middle-aged patients (40–50 years). While chemotherapy is more commonly proposed to elderly cancer patients, little is known about its impact on cognitive functioning. Among the published studies that have assessed the impact of ovarian cancer and its treatments on cognitive functioning, none focused on elderly patients.

Specificities of Elderly Cancer Patients

Aging is associated with cognitive and functional decline and comorbidities that may have a significant impact on the patient's autonomy. These alterations may be exacerbated by cancer and the toxicity of antitumoral agents, and functional decline is associated with a worse prognosis. Initial cognitive functioning and functional status could thus influence the choice of treatment.

The impact of cancer and chemotherapy on cognition and quality of life is thought to depend on several factors including baseline cognitive functioning, which is expected to be lower in older patients than in younger ones [32]. Little is known about the effect of treatment on the cognitive functioning of older patients [33] or whether chemotherapy-associated cognitive alterations affect an older patient's ability to perform daily activities.

Studies in Elderly Cancer Patients

Although there is no data available in ovarian cancer patients, the first longitudinal study on cognitive assessment in older patients with neuropsychological tests was conducted among breast cancer patients treated by adjuvant chemotherapy ($n=28$, mean age 71 ± 5) [33]. Thirty-nine percent of patients experienced a decline in cognitive performance within the 6 months following the start of chemotherapy (50 % had no change and 11 % improved). Furthermore, cancer survivors were also concerned by cognitive impairments: breast cancer survivors, who remained disease-free for more than one or two decades (mean age 73 ± 5.1 and 64 ± 6.4, respectively), performed worse on average than population controls [13, 34]. A similar pattern of differences in neuropsychological performances was found between groups to the detriment of the patient groups having undergone long-term chemotherapy. The impairment of executive functioning and psychomotor speed, working memory and attention, immediate and delayed verbal memory, and information processing speed [13] was in favor of dysfunctions involving the fronto-subcortical brain regions. Overall, the low number of studies performed in elderly patients suggests that cognitive disturbances affect the same functions as in younger patients. Previous cancer treatment may therefore exacerbate cognitive dysfunctions associated with age-related brain changes.

On the other hand, studies using cognitive screening tests like the Mini Mental State Examination or MMSE [35] did not find any cognitive impairment after cancer treatment. Cognitive impairments induced by cancer treatment are subtle and screening tests did not appear sensitive enough to detect them. However, even a small decline in elderly patients may have an important impact on their daily life.

Aging, Cognitive Decline, and Cancer

Many mechanisms are involved in cognitive deficits particularly in elderly cancer patients (Fig. 2.1 [36]). Aging, neurodegeneration, biological processes underlying cancer, the impact of cancer treatments, and cognitive decline appear to be linked, leading to the phase shift hypothesis, i.e., that cancer treatments may accelerate the aging process. According to this hypothesis, age-associated decline in cancer

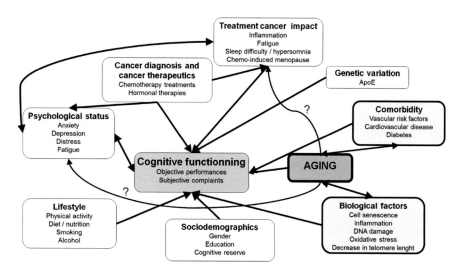

Fig. 2.1 Possible contributors to cognitive difficulties in elderly cancer patients (issued from Lange et al. [32], Cancer Treat Rev)

patients is not only parallel but is greater than that of older adults with no cancer history. An additional hypothesis, which does not exclude the latter, postulates that only vulnerable populations exhibit the accelerated aging pattern [5].

Some factors closely related to aging such as comorbidities (mainly cardiovascular disease, vascular risk factors, and diabetes), cognitive frailty, biological factors, tolerance to cancer treatment, and psychological status may contribute to exacerbating cognitive difficulties. Aging may potentially impact inflammation, oxidative stress, cell senescence, and DNA damage and lead to a decrease in telomere length, which may cause cognitive deficits [17, 37–40]. Physiological factors such as the patient's genetic makeup (e.g., the Apolipoprotein E (ApoE) associated with cognitive impairment related to Alzheimer's disease, brain trauma, and aging [41]), hormone levels, the inflammatory response to cancer treatments, postoperative cognitive dysfunctions, fatigue, and sleep difficulty or hypersomnia could also affect cognition. The patient's psychological status including degree of anxiety, depression, and stress increases vulnerability regarding cognitive function [42]. Lastly, it may be that other risk factors, such as low socioeconomic status, diet and nutrition, sedentary lifestyle, or alcohol and tobacco consumption, influence the development of both cancer and cognitive impairment [43]. However, the main cause of neuropsychological deficits in patients treated for cancer is chemotherapy [44].

Perspectives to Assess and Improve Cognition in Elderly Ovarian Cancer Patients

More than half of patients with ovarian cancer are over 65 at diagnosis [2]. Nevertheless, age is a risk factor for ovarian cancer and cognitive impairment. Unfortunately, the few studies assessing the impact of cancer and treatment among ovarian patients include very few patients over 65. Furthermore, these cancer patients usually had a general anesthesia of long duration, which could induce postoperative cognitive dysfunction, especially in elderly patients [45]. Moreover, the management of ovarian cancer includes multiple courses of chemotherapy, and a meta-analysis has shown that treatment of longer duration (i.e., the number of cycles of chemotherapy received) can lead to poorer cognitive performance [46].

While it is well established that chemotherapy induces cognitive impairment, there is emerging evidence suggesting that maintenance therapy with antiangiogenic agents plays a role in brain cognition and may induce neurotoxic effects on cognitive function [4, 47]. Some comorbidities, like hypertension, should be well controlled to limit the risk of cerebral toxicity.

Recommendations

Studies in elderly patients require a longitudinal design to assess cognition before any treatment insofar as these patients are more likely to exhibit age-related cognitive impairment before treatment compared to younger patients. Thus, future research should take into account the impact of chemotherapy and antiangiogenic treatment on cognition in order to better understand the trajectory of cognitive decline. Sufficient numbers of older patients and geriatric assessment of functional status should be included. Indeed, therapy-associated cognitive changes may affect an older patient's ability to perform daily activities. Cognitive assessment should also include batteries of neuropsychological tests rather than screening tests and should target cognitive domains hypothesized to be impacted by treatment, such as memory, executive functions, attention, and information processing speed. Such assessment should not be too long owing to the potential impact of fatigue in elderly patients [33].

In clinical practice, the comprehensive geriatric assessment (CGA) helps oncologists in the global care of elderly cancer patients. However, this multidimensional, multidisciplinary diagnostic instrument that aims to screen frail patients mainly assesses dependence, comorbidities, mood state, social support, and dementia. Cognition is assessed by screening tests like the MMSE [35], which is not sensitive enough to detect subtle disorders. As an alternative, the Montreal Cognitive Assessment (MOCA) [48], another quickly administered screening test, could be used because it is more sensitive to executive function impairments (11 items: visuospatial/executive, naming, memory, attention, language, abstraction, orientation; 10 min). When cognitive frailty is observed with the MOCA, a detailed cognitive evaluation could be added as an additional criterion in order to make the therapeutic decision. This is particularly justified if adjuvant chemotherapy is prescribed. Indeed, a diagnosis of cognitive deficit may alter the clinical decision concerning treatment [49].

Interventional Studies

Interventional research to treat cognitive changes is just emerging and includes both pharmacological and non-pharmacological approaches. Modafinil, a psychostimulant, has been reported in two studies to improve memory and attention and to reduce fatigue [50, 51]. Considering non-pharmacological approaches, e.g., cognitive rehabilitation, they have been shown to improve cognitive functioning [52, 53]. To date, however, only one study of cognitive rehabilitation has concerned elderly patients [54]. Physical exercise has also proved on cognitive function in cancer patients although such studies are limited and none has focused on elderly patients [55].

In summary, there is a growing body of evidence that cancer therapy may impact cognitive function although very few studies have concerned cognition in ovarian cancer patients despite the multiple courses of chemotherapy included in their management. Furthermore, no study has directly investigated elderly patients, even though age is a risk factor for ovarian cancer and cognitive impairment. Additional research is needed to apprehend the impact of cancer treatments on these women. Regarding oncologic practice, more detailed cognitive assessment of cognitively frail subjects would help oncologists to choose the most appropriate therapy.

References

1. Boykoff N, Moieni M, Subramanian SK. Confronting chemobrain: an in-depth look at survivors' reports of impact on work, social networks, and health care response. J Cancer Surviv. 2009;3:223–32.
2. Pignata S, Vermorken JB. Ovarian cancer in the elderly. Crit Rev Oncol Hematol. 2004;49:77–86.
3. Arriba LN, Fader AN, Frasure HE, von Gruenigen VE. A review of issues surrounding quality of life among women with ovarian cancer. Gynecol Oncol. 2010;119:390–6.
4. Ng T, Cheung YT, Ng QS, et al. Vascular endothelial growth factor inhibitors and cognitive impairment: evidence and controversies. Expert Opin Drug Saf. 2014;13:83–92.
5. Ahles TA, Root JC, Ryan EL. Cancer- and cancer treatment-associated cognitive change: an update on the state of the science. J Clin Oncol. 2012;30:3675–86.
6. Jim HS, Phillips KM, Chait S, et al. Meta-analysis of cognitive functioning in breast cancer survivors previously treated with standard-dose chemotherapy. J Clin Oncol. 2012;30:3578–87.
7. Kesler SR, Kent JS, O'Hara R. Prefrontal cortex and executive function impairments in primary breast cancer. Arch Neurol. 2011;68:1447–53.
8. Silverman DH, Dy CJ, Castellon SA, et al. Altered frontocortical, cerebellar, and basal ganglia activity in adjuvant-treated breast cancer survivors 5–10 years after chemotherapy. Breast Cancer Res Treat. 2007;103:303–11.
9. Joly F, Rigal O, Noal S, Giffard B. Cognitive dysfunction and cancer: which consequences in terms of disease management? Psychooncology. 2011;20:1251–8.
10. Shilling V, Jenkins V, Morris R, et al. The effects of adjuvant chemotherapy on cognition in women with breast cancer – preliminary results of an observational longitudinal study. Breast. 2005;14:142–50.
11. Wefel JS, Lenzi R, Theriault RL, et al. The cognitive sequelae of standard-dose adjuvant chemotherapy in women with breast carcinoma: results of a prospective, randomized, longitudinal trial. Cancer. 2004;100:2292–9.
12. Ahles TA, Saykin AJ, Furstenberg CT, et al. Neuropsychologic impact of standard-dose systemic chemotherapy in long-term survivors of breast cancer and lymphoma. J Clin Oncol. 2002;20:485–93.
13. Koppelmans V, Breteler MM, Boogerd W, et al. Neuropsychological performance in survivors of breast cancer more than 20 years after adjuvant chemotherapy. J Clin Oncol. 2012;30:1080–6.
14. Koppelmans V, Breteler MM, Boogerd W, et al. Late effects of adjuvant chemotherapy for adult onset non-CNS cancer; cognitive impairment, brain structure and risk of dementia. Crit Rev Oncol Hematol. 2013;88:87–101.
15. Ahles TA. Brain vulnerability to chemotherapy toxicities. Psychooncology. 2012;21:1141–8.
16. Scherling CS, Smith A. Opening up the window into "chemobrain": a neuroimaging review. Sensors (Basel). 2013;13:3169–203.
17. Ahles TA, Saykin AJ. Candidate mechanisms for chemotherapy-induced cognitive changes. Nat Rev Cancer. 2007;7:192–201.
18. Hutchinson AD, Hosking JR, Kichenadasse G, et al. Objective and subjective cognitive impairment following chemotherapy for cancer: a systematic review. Cancer Treat Rev. 2012;38:926–34.
19. Pullens MJ, de Vries J, Roukema JA. Subjective cognitive dysfunction in breast cancer patients: a systematic review. Psychooncology. 2010;19:1127–38.
20. Hensley ML, Correa DD, Thaler H, et al. Phase I/II study of weekly paclitaxel plus carboplatin and gemcitabine as first-line treatment of advanced-stage ovarian cancer: pathologic complete response and longitudinal assessment of impact on cognitive functioning. Gynecol Oncol. 2006;102:270–7.
21. Mehnert A, Scherwath A, Schirmer L, et al. The association between neuropsychological impairment, self-perceived cognitive deficits, fatigue and health related quality of life in breast

cancer survivors following standard adjuvant versus high-dose chemotherapy. Patient Educ Couns. 2007;66:108–18.
22. Correa DD, Hess LM. Cognitive function and quality of life in ovarian cancer. Gynecol Oncol. 2012;124:404–9.
23. Briones TL, Woods J. Chemotherapy-induced cognitive impairment is associated with decreases in cell proliferation and histone modifications. BMC Neurosci. 2011;12:124.
24. Gangloff A, Hsueh WA, Kesner AL, et al. Estimation of paclitaxel biodistribution and uptake in human-derived xenografts in vivo with (18)F-fluoropaclitaxel. J Nucl Med. 2005;46:1866–71.
25. Abbas O, Shamseddin A, Temraz S, Haydar A. Posterior reversible encephalopathy syndrome after bevacizumab therapy in a normotensive patient. BMJ Case Rep. 2013;2013:bcr2012007995.
26. van der Veldt AA, van den Eertwegh AJ, Hoekman K, et al. Reversible cognitive disorders after sunitinib for advanced renal cell cancer in patients with preexisting arteriosclerotic leukoencephalopathy. Ann Oncol. 2007;18:1747–50.
27. Mayerhofer K, Bodner-Adler B, Bodner K, et al. A paclitaxel-containing chemotherapy does not cause central nervous adverse effects: a prospective study in patients with ovarian cancer. Anticancer Res. 2000;20:4051–5.
28. Hess LM, Chambers SK, Hatch K, et al. Pilot study of the prospective identification of changes in cognitive function during chemotherapy treatment for advanced ovarian cancer. J Support Oncol. 2010;8:252–8.
29. Correa DD, Zhou Q, Thaler HT, et al. Cognitive functions in long-term survivors of ovarian cancer. Gynecol Oncol. 2010;119:366–9.
30. Wagner L, Sweet J, Butt Z, et al. Measuring patient self-reported cognitive function: development of the Functional Assessment of Cancer Therapy–Cognitive Function instrument. J Support Oncol. 2009;7:w32–9.
31. Wefel JS, Vardy J, Ahles T, Schagen SB. International Cognition and Cancer Task Force recommendations to harmonise studies of cognitive function in patients with cancer. Lancet Oncol. 2011;12:703–8.
32. Lange M, Rigal O, Clarisse B, et al. Cognitive dysfunctions in elderly cancer patients: a new challenge for oncologists. Cancer Treat Rev. 2014;40:810–7.
33. Hurria A, Rosen C, Hudis C, et al. Cognitive function of older patients receiving adjuvant chemotherapy for breast cancer: a pilot prospective longitudinal study. J Am Geriatr Soc. 2006;54:925–31.
34. Yamada TH, Denburg NL, Beglinger LJ, Schultz SK. Neuropsychological outcomes of older breast cancer survivors: cognitive features ten or more years after chemotherapy. J Neuropsychiatry Clin Neurosci. 2010;22:48–54.
35. Folstein MF, Folstein SE, Mchugh PR. Mini-mental state. A practical method for grading the cognitive state of patients for the clinician. J Psychiatr Res. 1975;12:189–98.
36. Mandelblatt JS, Hurria A, Mcdonald BC, et al. Cognitive effects of cancer and its treatments at the intersection of aging: what do we know; what do we need to know? Semin Oncol. 2013;40:709–25.
37. Ahles TA, Saykin AJ, Noll WW, et al. The relationship of APOE genotype to neuropsychological performance in long-term cancer survivors treated with standard dose chemotherapy. Psychooncology. 2003;12:612–9.
38. Johnson T, Monk T, Rasmussen LS, et al. Postoperative cognitive dysfunction in middle-aged patients. Anesthesiology. 2002;96:1351–7.
39. Meyers CA, Albitar M, Estey E. Cognitive impairment, fatigue, and cytokine levels in patients with acute myelogenous leukemia or myelodysplastic syndrome. Cancer. 2005;104:788–93.
40. Reichenberg A, Yirmiya R, Schuld A, et al. Cytokine-associated emotional and cognitive disturbances in humans. Arch Gen Psychiatry. 2001;58:445–52.
41. Strittmatter WJ, Saunders AM, Schmechel D, et al. Apolipoprotein E: high-avidity binding to beta-amyloid and increased frequency of type 4 allele in late-onset familial Alzheimer disease. Proc Natl Acad Sci U S A. 1993;90:1977–81.

42. Giffard B, Viard A, Dayan J, et al. Autobiographical memory, self, and stress-related psychiatric disorders: which implications in cancer patients? Neuropsychol Rev. 2013;23:157–68.
43. Alzheimer's Association. Adopt a brain-healthy diet. 2012.
44. Vardy J, Wefel JS, Ahles T, et al. Cancer and cancer-therapy related cognitive dysfunction: an international perspective from the Venice cognitive workshop. Ann Oncol. 2008;19:623–9.
45. Monk TG, Weldon BC, Garvan CW, et al. Predictors of cognitive dysfunction after major noncardiac surgery. Anesthesiology. 2008;108:18–30.
46. Hodgson KD, Hutchinson AD, Wilson CJ, Nettelbeck T. A meta-analysis of the effects of chemotherapy on cognition in patients with cancer. Cancer Treat Rev. 2013;39:297–304.
47. Mulder SF, Bertens D, Desar IM, et al. Impairment of cognitive functioning during Sunitinib or Sorafenib treatment in cancer patients: a cross sectional study. BMC Cancer. 2014;14:219.
48. Nasreddine ZS, Phillips NA, Bedirian V, et al. The Montreal Cognitive Assessment, MoCA: a brief screening tool for mild cognitive impairment. J Am Geriatr Soc. 2005;53:695–9.
49. Pal SK, Katheria V, Hurria A. Evaluating the older patient with cancer: understanding frailty and the geriatric assessment. CA Cancer J Clin. 2010;60:120–32.
50. Lundorff LE, Jonsson BH, Sjogren P. Modafinil for attentional and psychomotor dysfunction in advanced cancer: a double-blind, randomised, cross-over trial. Palliat Med. 2009;23:731–8.
51. Kohli S, Fisher SG, Tra Y, et al. The effect of modafinil on cognitive function in breast cancer survivors. Cancer. 2009;115:2605–16.
52. Schuurs A, Green HJ. A feasibility study of group cognitive rehabilitation for cancer survivors: enhancing cognitive function and quality of life. Psychooncology. 2013;22:1043–9.
53. Von Ah D, Carpenter JS, Saykin A, et al. Advanced cognitive training for breast cancer survivors: a randomized controlled trial. Breast Cancer Res Treat. 2012;135:799–809.
54. Mcdougall GJ, Becker H, Acee TW, et al. Symptom management of affective and cognitive disturbance with a group of cancer survivors. Arch Psychiatr Nurs. 2011;25:24–35.
55. Von Ah D, Storey S, Jansen CE, Allen DH. Coping strategies and interventions for cognitive changes in patients with cancer. Semin Oncol Nurs. 2013;29:288–99.

Histopathology of Ovarian Cancers in Elderly Patients

3

Mojgan Devouassoux-Shisheboran

Contents

Introduction

According to 2014 WHO classification [1] and based on their morphology, primary ovarian tumors are subdivided into three large categories; epithelial (60 %), germ cell (30 %), and sex-cord stromal tumors (8 %). However, malignant ovarian tumors are in their vast majority (80–85 %) of epithelial type called carcinomas. Malignant germ cell and sex-cord stromal tumors comprise approximately 10 % of all ovarian cancers. Also, about 5–14 % of cancers are metastatic tumors to the ovaries. Ovarian tumors account for a considerable proportion of clinically important neoplasms in the female, with a very wide range of age from infant to elderly patients. About two

M. Devouassoux-Shisheboran, MD, PhD (✉)
Department of Pathology, Hôpital de la Croix Rousse, 69317 Lyon Cedex 04, France
e-mail: mojgan.devouassoux@chu-lyon.fr

© Springer International Publishing Switzerland 2016
G. Freyer (ed.), *Ovarian Cancer in Elderly Patients*,
DOI 10.1007/978-3-319-23588-2_3

thirds of ovarian tumors occur in women in the reproductive age group and 80–90 % of them in women between 20 and 65 years, while less than 5 % are seen in children. Around 75–80 % of ovarian tumors are benign, and 55–65 % of benign tumors occur in young ladies under 40 years. In contrast, 80–90 % of ovarian carcinomas are detected after the age of 40 years and 30–40 % of them after the age of 65 years. The age-specific incidence of ovarian epithelial cancer rises from 20 to 80 years and subsequently declines. The chance that a primary ovarian epithelial tumors is of borderline or invasive malignancy in a patient under the age of 40 years is approximately 1 in 10, while beyond that age it rises to 1 in 3 [2].

Ovarian Carcinomas

Ovarian epithelial tumors are subclassified into several categories according to two criteria: (1) the degree of epithelial proliferation and invasion and (2) the type of epithelium composing the tumor.

Benign epithelial tumors (adenoma and cystadenoma) are characterized by the absence of cell proliferation and invasion. They represent 60 % of all epithelial tumors. They can occur at any age but are most often seen in adults and 60 % under the age of 40 years.

Borderline tumors are characterized by cell proliferation and a minor degree of nuclear atypia without stromal invasion. They represent 10 % of all epithelial tumors. They occur at a slightly younger age than carcinoma (mean 45 years).

Carcinomas are characterized by both cell proliferations, nuclear atypia and stromal invasion. They represent 30 % of all epithelial tumors and 80–85 % of all ovarian cancers. They are mostly seen in elderly patients with a mean age of 60 years.

Ovarian carcinomas represent a heterogeneous group that differs in their morphology, molecular biology, pathogenesis, and behavior. Their classification was initially based on the morphology of the type of epithelium composing the tumor. However, new findings in genetics were ended by a real phenotypic-genotypic classification of these tumors that represent five distinct diseases [3] (Table 3.1).

Serous Carcinomas

Serous carcinomas represent the vast majority of primary ovarian malignant tumors (75–80 %) and are composed of columnar cells with cilia. They are subdivided into high-grade and low-grade serous carcinomas [1, 4].

High-grade serous carcinomas (HGSC) account for 85–90 % of serous carcinomas and 70 % of ovarian surface epithelial carcinomas. This is the ovarian carcinoma subtype that most people have in mind when talking about "ovarian cancer" and account for most deaths due to ovarian cancer. HGSC is a disease of elderly patients with a mean age of 64 years. This carcinoma is bilateral in 60 % of cases and is detected in advanced stage in more than 80 % of cases. HGSC is very large cystic and solid tumor with frequent areas of hemorrhage and necrosis.

Table 3.1 Phenotypic-genotypic classification of ovarian carcinomas: five distinct diseases according to Prat [3]

	HG serous	LG serous	Mucinous	Endometrioid	Clear cell
Incidence	70 %	<5 %	3 %	10 %	5–10 %
Risk factors	BRCA1/2	?	?	HNPCC	HNPCC+/-
Precursor lesions	STIC	Borderline serous	Borderline mucinous	endometriosis	endometriosis
Molecular abnormalities	P53/BRCA	BRAF KRAS	KRAS HER2	PTEN ARID1A	HNF1b ARID1A PIK3CA MET
Pattern of spread	Very early transcoelomic	Trans coelomic	Usually confined to ovary	Usually confined to pelvis	Usually confined to pelvis
Chemosensitivity	High	Intermediate	Low	High	Low
Prognosis	Poor	Intermediate	Favorable	Favorable	Intermediate

Morphologically, the cells form papillae, solid masses, or slit-like spaces with high-grade nuclear atypia and more than 12 mitoses per 10 high-power fields. Immunohistochemical findings show CK7, PAX8, and WT1 positivity, while CK20 is negative. HGSC show *TP53* mutation in more than 96 % of cases with protein overexpression detected by immunohistochemical analyses. *Transitional cell carcinoma* is a rare variant of ovarian high-grade carcinoma (3 %) showing a papillary pattern seen in urothelial carcinomas. Most tumors show an admixture of HGSC. They have the same immunoprofile than HGSC; thus, the new WHO classification considers this type of carcinoma to be a variant of HGSC [1]. HGSC are genomically instable and aneuploid. Around 10 % of patients with HGSC have a germ line *BRCA1* or *BRCA2* mutations. Moreover, sporadic tumors show BRCAness phenotype with BRCA loss by somatic mutation (3 %) or promoter hypermethylation (11 %) of *BRCA* genes [5]. HGSC were thought to drive from surface epithelium without a known precursor according to incessant ovulation theory. However, pathological studies on prophylactic bilateral salpingo-oophorectomies in patients with germ line *BRCA* mutations have demonstrated occult intraepithelial serous carcinomas in 17 % of cases, mostly located in the fimbriated end of the fallopian tube [6]. This serous tubal intraepithelial carcinoma (STIC) showed the same *TP53* mutation profile than invasive ovarian carcinoma in patients with *BRCA* mutation, indicating that it might represent the precursor of ovarian serous carcinomas. STIC was also detected in 60 % of sporadic ovarian and peritoneal carcinomas with the same *TP53* mutational profile [7], in favor of a direct relationship between a noninvasive lesion in the fallopian tube and an invasive carcinoma in the ovary or the peritoneum.

Low-grade serous carcinoma (LGSC) is less common, representing 10–15 % of serous carcinomas and <5 % of all ovarian carcinomas. It occurs at a younger age than HGSC (mean 43 versus 64 years). It is associated with a serous borderline tumor (60 %) or represents the recurrent lesion seen after a diagnosis of borderline serous tumor (75 %). It is composed of papillae or micropapillae without nuclear atypia and with few mitoses. They are slow-growing tumors with 10-year survival rate of 50 % (overall survival 82 months) and a relative insensitivity to chemotherapy. LGSC's immunoprofile is comparable to HGSC, but there is no *TP53* mutation in these tumors, so there is no P53 overexpression by immunohistochemistry. LGSC are genetically stable and diploid tumors [8]. They show *KRAS* (mutation exon 12 % or 13 % in 19 % of cases), *BRAF* mutation V600E (5–38 %), or *ERBB2* mutation (6 % of cases) that are mutually exclusive [9, 10]. It has however been shown that *BRAF* mutation (V600E) is more frequent in serous borderline tumors (28–48 %) as compared to LGSC (5–38 %) [11, 12].

Endometrioid Carcinomas

Endometrioid carcinomas account for 10 % of all ovarian carcinomas and are mostly unilateral (60 %) solid masses with smooth outer surface. They are composed of glands resembling endometrial epithelium and may be associated (23–42 %) with ovarian or pelvic endometriosis. They show CK7, PAX8, hormone receptor (estrogen and progesterone) positivity and are WT1 and CK20 negative, helping in their distinction from serous and colonic carcinomas, respectively. They are graded into three grades according to the FIGO system, based on the presence of solid areas and the nuclear atypia. Grade 3 tumors tend to show *TP53* mutations and may be difficult to distinguish from HGSC. Genotypically, endometrioid carcinomas show molecular abnormalities seen in their endometrial counterpart with *CTNNB-1*(48 %), *PIK3CA* (20 %), *PTEN* (20 %), and *ARID1A* (30 %) mutations. These tumors are the subtype of ovarian carcinomas most often seen in patients with LYNCH syndrome. Sporadic cases also show microsatellite instabilities (hypermethylation of *MLH1* promoter) in a number of cases [13, 14]. The same mutations (*PTEN* and *ARID1A*) have been detected in the carcinoma and adjacent endometriosis cysts, indicating that endometriosis might be the precursor for endometrioid ovarian carcinomas.

Also, *pure endometrioid mesenchymal* and *mixed epithelial/mesenchymal tumors*, reminiscent of those seen in the uterine corpus, are seldom encountered in the ovary.

Pure endometrioid mesenchymal tumors are subdivided into low-grade and high-grade endometrioid stromal sarcomas and are rare tumors occurring during the fifth and sixth decade of life. They have the same morphology and immunoprofile than their uterine counterpart and may arise in the ovary from endometriosis. A uterine tumor should be ruled out before making a diagnosis of primary ovarian endometrioid stromal sarcoma.

Mixed epithelial/mesenchymal tumors are biphasic tumors with a sarcomatous component and a benign or malignant epithelial component. The latter is used to subdivide these mixed tumors into adenosarcomas and carcinosarcomas (malignant mixed mullerian tumor/MMMT) (see also below), respectively. MMMT is a tumor of elderly women seen usually in patients over 60 years old. It is a very high-grade and aggressive neoplasm, often detected at a high stage with extra-ovarian spread and a median survival of less than 24 months [15]. The epithelial component is usually of high-grade serous, endometrioid, and/or clear cell carcinoma. The sarcomatous component may be homologous or heterologous with rhabdomyosarcoma, chondro- or osteo- or liposarcomatous elements.

Mucinous Carcinomas

Primary mucinous carcinomas are of intestinal type (containing goblet cells) and comprise only 2–3 % of ovarian carcinomas. They are unilateral, stage I (75–80 %), large (18–22 cm), and multicystic tumors filled with mucus. They often contain solid areas. Histologically, they are composed of cysts and glands of varying size, with a confluent pattern and back-to-back glands. Complex papillary architecture is also seen. The cells are tall, columnar, and stratified with basophilic cytoplasm containing mucin. Invasive mucinous carcinomas are subclassified into expansile and infiltrative type. *The expansile-type mucinous carcinomas* are stage I disease with a very good prognosis and are composed of confluent glands and a papillary pattern, seen mostly in younger patients. *Infiltrative-type mucinous carcinomas* have a destructive invasion pattern with desmoplastic stromal reaction and are more likely to have extra-ovarian spread [16, 17]. Mucinous adenocarcinomas may be graded according to their nuclear features [18]. On immunohistochemical study, ovarian mucinous carcinomas show diffuse CK7 positivity, while CK20 is usually less diffusely positive. Hormone receptors (estrogen and progesterone), WT1, and PAX8, are usually negative. Mucinous carcinomas arise from a mucinous borderline tumor. Thus, mucinous ovarian tumors show often a heterogeneous pattern with coexisting areas of mucinous cystadenoma, mucinous borderline tumor, and mucinous adenocarcinoma. Their diagnosis requires a thorough sampling with 2 blocks per cm of tumor.

The major difficulty in the diagnosis of mucinous ovarian tumor is their distinction from a metastasis from gastrointestinal or pancreatobiliary tract tumor. The bilaterality, a multinodular pattern in the ovary, a small size (usually less than 10 cm), ovarian surface involvement, and a massive disorganized pattern of invasion are characteristics seen in metastatic tumors. Appendicectomy and a clinical assessment of the gastrointestinal tract is useful in case of a mucinous carcinoma in the ovary.

Molecular biology in mucinous ovarian carcinoma shows *KRAS* mutations codons 12 and/or 13 in 68–86 % of cases. An identical mutational profile in different areas from benign (55 %) to borderline (73 %) and malignant (86 %) of the same tumor in 12/15 cases supports the morphological continuum of tumor progression in ovarian mucinous tumors [19]. Amplification of *HER2* gene has been shown in 18 % of carcinomas and 6 % of borderline tumors. *HER2* amplification and *KRAS* mutation are mutually exclusive (5.6 % show both abnormalities). *HER2* amplification or *KRAS* mutation seem to be associated with decreased in recurrence and death when compared with double-negative tumors (34 %) [20]

Sero-Mucinous Carcinomas

This variant has been added to the new WHO classification 2014 [1], while it was described as endocervical mucinous carcinoma in the previous WHO classification 2003. Morphologically, this rare variant of ovarian carcinoma is composed of a mixture of serous- and endocervical-type mucinous cells with foci of endometrioid and squamous differentiation. The mean age is 45 years and it is seldom seen in elderly patients. This tumor is often associated with endometriosis that may represent its precursor. When stage I, the tumor has a good prognosis, while half of patients with advanced disease died because of their tumor [21]

Clear Cell Carcinomas

Clear cell carcinomas (CCC) represent 6 % of all ovarian carcinomas in western countries but 15–25 % of carcinomas in Japan. They are most often diagnosed at low stage (I/II) (49 % versus 17 % for HGSC). They occur at a younger age than HGSC (55 years versus 64 years). Less than 10 % of cases are seen in the fourth decade, and most patients are 50–70 years old. They seem to have a worst prognosis with 5-year survival rate of 60 % versus 80 % for HGSC. However, when looking at stage I disease only, the prognosis is similar to HGSC at the same stage (85 % versus 86 % for HGSC). CCC show a low response to platinum/taxane therapy (11–45 %) [22].

The majority (99 %) of ovarian clear cell tumors are carcinomas and clear cell adenofibromas or borderline tumors are exceptional lesions (<1 %). The tumor is predominantly solid and unilateral (98 % of stage I cases), with a yellow cut surface. The tumor is composed of papillae with a hyalinized core and solid, tubulo-cystic, and glandular pattern. The cells are large with a clear or eosinophilic cytoplasm. The nuclei are pleomorphic, irregular, and hyperchromatic, but the mitotic index might be lower than what one could expect from the nuclear atypia.

The immunohistochemical study shows diffuse CK7 positivity but CK20, hormone receptors (estrogen and progesterone), and WT1 are negative. HNF1beta (hepatocyte nuclear factor) has been shown to be positive in 93 % of ovarian CCC versus 2 % of non-clear cell ovarian carcinomas [23]. Napsin A is also positive in 83% of ovarian clear cell carcinomas, while serous, endometrioid and mucinous carcinomas are usually negative. There is no *TP53* mutation. CCC is associated with ovarian or pelvic endometriosis in 21–54 % of cases. Exomic sequences in 8 cases after immunoaffinity purification of cancer cells has shown four mutated genes in at least two tumors: *ARID1A, PIK3CA, KRAS,* and *PPP2R1A* [24].

Somatic truncating or missense mutations in *ARID1A* (the AT-rich interactive domain 1A [SSWI-like] gene) encoding BAF250 (a key component of the SWI-SNF chromatin remodeling complex) have been found in 46 % of 119 clear cell carcinomas, 30 % of 33 endometrioid carcinomas, and none of 76 HGSC. The same mutation was also seen in 2 endometriotic cysts adjacent to tumor, indicating that endometriosis might be the precursor of ovarian CCC [25]. Activating mutations in *PIK3CA* gene exon 20 (H1047R in the kinase domain) has been seen in 33–43 % CCC and 90 % of associated endometriotic cysts [26]. Overexpression (complete membrane staining with moderate to strong intensity in >10 % cells) and amplification (≥4 copies in ≥40 % cells) of *MET* gene are reported in 22 % and 24 % CCC, respectively, while non-CCC show 0 % and 3 % overexpression or amplification of this gene. Moreover, *MET* overexpression has been identified as an independent unfavorable prognostic factor with 5-year survival of 33 % for overexpressed MET cases versus 76 % for MET-negative patients [27].

Malignant Brenner Tumors

This is a rare variant of ovarian low-grade carcinoma (<5 % of all ovarian Brenner tumors) showing an admixture of benign or borderline Brenner tumor and malignant urothelial-type cell carcinomas. These tumors occur in women over 50 years of age. *PIK3CA* mutations (exon 9) have been shown, but in contrast to transitional cell carcinomas, they don't present *TP53* mutations. Most tumors are stage I and have an excellent prognosis with 88 % 5-year survival rate. When extra-ovarian, the prognosis is similar to other ovarian carcinomas [28].

Undifferentiated Carcinomas

This type of carcinoma represents less than 1 % of cases. It is a high-grade tumor with sheets of small or large cells with pleomorphic nuclei and high mitotic index. The positivity of epithelial markers although scant (pancytokeratin, CK7, CK18, EMA) helps in distinguishing them from lymphomas, melanomas, or sarcomas. Undifferentiated carcinomas occurring in elderly patients should not be confused with small cell carcinoma, hypercalcemic type that is usually seen in young patients between 9 and 43 years old and shows typical follicle-like spaces.

Malignant Mixed Mesodermal Tumor (Carcinosarcoma) (MMMT)

MMMT accounts for less than 1 % of ovarian cancers. It is essentially seen in elderly patients with a mean age of 65 years. Three quarters of them are seen between 60 and 80 years. These tumors are large cystic and solid with massive areas of hemorrhage and necrosis and are often seen at an advance stage with peritoneal spread (75 %). They are composed of a mixture of high-grade epithelial component with grade 3 endometrioid, clear cell, and high-grade serous carcinomas and a high-grade stromal component usually with hyperchromatic round or spindle cells showing many mitoses. Heterologous elements in the form of rhabdomyosarcomatous, osteosarcomatous, chondrosarcomatous, or liposarcomatous elements may be seen. MMMT has a very poor prognosis with the overall 5-year survival of <30 % [29].

Ovarian Germ Cell Tumors

This category of ovarian tumors accounts for 30 % of ovarian tumors but over 95 % of them are mature teratomas (dermoid cyst). Malignant germ cell tumors are rare (2–3 %) and are usually seen in patients less than 20 years old. One of the malignant germ cell tumors that can be seen in elderly patients is a mature teratoma with secondary malignant tumors. Around 1–2 % of mature teratomas contain a cancer of adult type, in the form of carcinoma, essentially squamous cell carcinoma (80 %) or adenocarcinoma (7 %). Sarcomas may also be seen. The mean age of patients is 59 years. If a women 70 years of age or older has a dermoid cyst, there is an approximately 15 % chance that it will contain a secondary malignant tumor [30]. Grossly, the dermoid cyst contains a solid, white area, corresponding to the malignant transformation of a teratomatous component.

Ovarian Sex-Cord Stromal Tumors

This category accounts for 8 % of ovarian tumors.

Pure stromal tumors represent the majority of cases (87 %) and are mostly benign (fibroma, thecoma, sclerosing stromal tumors, signet-ring and microcystic stromal tumors). The malignant tumor of this category is fibrosarcoma that is seen in older patients (42–73 years, average 58 years). Fibrosarcoma is a large, unilateral, solid tumor with areas of hemorrhage and necrosis. It is composed of spindle cells with moderate to severe atypia and more than 4 mitoses per ten high-power fields [31]. Cellular fibroma without nuclear atypia showing more than 4 mitoses per ten high-power fields has been called mitotically active cellular fibroma with a potential for local recurrences but with no metastatic disease [32]. Ovarian fibrosarcomas are aggressive neoplasms with recurrences and metastases and a mortality rate of 66 % [31]. Some steroid cell tumors may have a malignant behavior when showing features such as size >7 cm, >2 mitoses per 10 high-power fields, necrosis, and nuclear atypia.

Sex-cord tumors are subdivided into different tumors including granulosa cell tumors (GCT) (12 %) and Sertoli-Leydig cell tumors (<0.5 %). The later are mixed sex-cord tumors and are seen in young patients averaging 25 years. The former are pure sex-cord tumors that are of two types, juvenile GCT (5 % of cases) seen in the first three decades of life and adult GCT (95 %) encountered in postmenopausal ladies between 50 and 55 years. This is a hormone-secreting tumor and the majority of patients present with estrogenic manifestations and postmenopausal bleeding. Around 5 % of patients have either endometrial hyperplasia or adenocarcinoma (endometrioid-type low grade). Adult GCT account for 1–2 % of all ovarian neoplasms. It is a large (average 12 cm), solid and cystic, unilateral (90 %) tumor. Rarely, the tumor may be entirely cystic. The cut surface is white to yellow. The tumor is composed of small cells with scant cytoplasm and ovoid or angular nuclei showing longitudinal groove ("coffee bean"). Nuclear pleomorphism may rarely be seen. The mitotic activity is usually low. The cells form insular, trabecular, tubular pattern. The characteristic architecture is microfollicular with "Call-Exner bodies." The stroma between cells is fibromatous. An immunohistochemical study shows a perinuclear staining pattern with cytokeratin but EMA is negative. Sex-cord markers (inhibin, calretinin, FOXL2) are usually expressed. Recently, a missense somatic mutation in *FOXL2* gene affecting codon 134 has been reported in 95 % of adult GCT, few thecoma, and few juvenile GCT but not in other types of ovarian tumors [33].

Most adult granulosa cell tumor are stage I disease at diagnosis. However, adult granulosa cell tumors have a malignant potential and can recur (locally in the pelvis or distant metastases in the liver, spleen, lung) (20–30 %) after 5 to more than 20 years after the diagnosis. The stage is the most important prognostic factor (10 years' survival rate of 86 % for stage I versus 49 % for stages II–IV). The only prognostic factor influencing the recurrences for stage I tumors seems to be tumor rupture with an overall survival rate of 86–100 % for stage IA versus 60 % for stage IC [34]. The number of mitosis, nuclear atypia, age over 40 years, and tumor size over 6 cm have also been reported to be responsible for unfavorable outcome but seem not to be significatively important features.

Conclusion

Ovarian cancer is a heterogeneous group of lesions, with specific morphology, biology, response to treatment, and behavior. The correct diagnosis is based on histopathological examination of the specimen. In elderly patients with ascites, cytology may help in making the diagnosis of malignancy with a good accuracy (60 % of sensitivity and 100 % of specificity) but the cytology won't be able to distinguish between the different subtypes of carcinomas. In inoperable tumors a percutaneous US or CT-guided peritoneal fine-needle biopsy may be an alternative to have tissue material for correct morphological and biological analyses for near-future personalized medicine.

References

1. Kurman RJ, Carcangiu ML, Herrington CS, Young RH. WHO classification of tumours of female reproductive organs. Lyon: IARC Press; 2014.
2. Yancik R, Ries LG, Yates JW. Ovarian cancer in the elderly: an analysis of Surveillance, Epidemiology, and End Results Program data. Am J Obstet Gynecol. 1986;154:639–47.
3. Prat J. New insights into ovarian cancer pathology. Ann Oncol. 2012;23:111–7.
4. Malpica A, Deavers MT, Lu K, Bodurka DC, Atkinson EN, Gershenson DM, Silva EG. Grading ovarian serous carcinoma using a two-tier system. Am J Surg Pathol. 2004;28:496–504.
5. The Cancer Genome Atlas Research Network. Integrated genomic analyses of ovarian carcinoma. Nature. 2011;474:609–15.
6. Lee Y, Miron A, Drapkin R, Nucci MR, Medeiros F, Saleemuddin A, Garber J, Birch C, Mou H, Gordon RW, Cramer DW, McKeon FD, Crum CP. A candidate precursor to serous carcinoma that originates in the distal fallopian tube. J Pathol. 2007;211:26–35.
7. Przybycin CG, Kurman RJ, Ronnett BM, Shih IM, Vang R. Are all pelvic (nonuterine) serous carcinomas of tubal origin? Am J Surg Pathol. 2010;34:1407–16.
8. Jones S, Wang TL, Kurman RJ, Nakayama K, Velculescu VE, Vogelstein B, Kinzler KW, Papadopoulos N, Shih IM. Low-grade serous carcinomas of the ovary contain very few point mutations. J Pathol. 2012;226:413–20.
9. Anglesio MS, Arnold JM, George J, Tinker AV, Tothill R, Waddell N, Simms L, Locandro B, Fereday S, Traficante N, Russell P, Sharma R, Birrer MJ; AOCS Study Group, deFazio A, Chenevix-Trench G, Bowtell DD. Mutation of ERBB2 provides a novel alternative mechanism for the ubiquitous activation of RAS-MAPK in ovarian serous low malignant potential tumors. Mol Cancer Res. 2008;6:1678–90.
10. Romero I, Sun CC, Wong KK, Bast Jr RC, Gershenson DM. Low-grade serous carcinoma: new concepts and emerging therapies. Gynecol Oncol. 2013;130:660–6.
11. Grisham RN, Iyer G, Garg K, DeLair D, Hyman DM, Zhou Q, Iasonos A, Berger MF, Dao F, Spriggs DR, Levine DA, Aghajanian C, Solit DB. BRAF mutation is associated with early stage disease and improved outcome in patients with low-grade serous ovarian cancer. Cancer. 2013;119:548–54.
12. Wong KK, Tsang YT, Deavers MT, Mok SC, Zu Z, Sun C, Malpica A, Wolf JK, Lu KH, Gershenson DM. BRAF mutation is rare in advanced-stage low-grade ovarian serous carcinomas. Am J Pathol. 2010;177:1611–7.
13. Sato N, Tsunoda H, Nishida M, Morishita Y, Takimoto Y, Kubo T, Noguchi M. Loss of heterozygosity on 10q23.3 and mutation of the tumor suppressor gene PTEN in benign endometrial cyst of the ovary: possible sequence progression from benign endometrial cyst to endometrioid carcinoma and clear cell carcinoma of the ovary. Cancer Res. 2000;60:7052–6.

14. Geyer JT, López-García MA, Sánchez-Estevez C, Sarrió D, Moreno-Bueno G, Franceschetti I, Palacios J, Oliva E. Pathogenetic pathways in ovarian endometrioid adenocarcinoma: a molecular study of 29 cases. Am J Surg Pathol. 2009;33:1157–63.
15. Brown E, Stewart M, Rye T, Al-Nafussi A, Williams AR, Bradburn M, Smyth J, Gabra H. Carcinosarcoma of the ovary: 19 years of prospective data from a single center. Cancer. 2004;100:2148–53.
16. Lee KR, Scully RE. Mucinous tumors of the ovary: a clinicopathologic study of 196 borderline tumors (of intestinal type) and carcinomas, including an evaluation of 11 cases with 'pseudomyxoma peritonei'. Am J Surg Pathol. 2000;24:1447–64.
17. Hoerl HD, Hart WR. Primary ovarian mucinous cystadenocarcinomas: a clinicopathologic study of 49 cases with long-term follow-up. Am J Surg Pathol. 1998;22:1449–62.
18. Rodríguez IM, Prat J. Mucinous tumors of the ovary: a clinicopathologic analysis of 75 borderline tumors (of intestinal type) and carcinomas. Am J Surg Pathol. 2002;26:139–52.
19. Cuatrecasas M, Villanueva A, Matias-Guiu X, Prat J. K-ras mutations in mucinous ovarian tumors: a clinicopathologic and molecular study of 95 cases. Cancer. 1997;79:1581–6.
20. Anglesio MS, Kommoss S, Tolcher MC, Clarke B, Galletta L, Porter H, Damaraju S, Fereday S, Winterhoff BJ, Kalloger SE, Senz J, Yang W, Steed H, Allo G, Ferguson S, Shaw P, Teoman A, Garcia JJ, Schoolmeester JK, Bakkum-Gamez J, Tinker AV, Bowtell DD, Huntsman DG, Gilks CB, McAlpine JN. Molecular characterization of mucinous ovarian tumours supports a stratified treatment approach with HER2 targeting in 19% of carcinomas. J Pathol. 2013;229:111–20.
21. Shappell HW, Riopel MA, Smith Sehdev AE, Ronnett BM, Kurman RJ. Diagnostic criteria and behavior of ovarian seromucinous (endocervical-type mucinous and mixed cell-type) tumors: atypical proliferative (borderline) tumors, intraepithelial, microinvasive, and invasive carcinomas. Am J Surg Pathol. 2002;26:1529–41.
22. Anglesio MS, Carey MS, Köbel M, Mackay H, Huntsman DG, Vancouver Ovarian Clear Cell Symposium Speakers. Clear cell carcinoma of the ovary: a report from the first Ovarian Clear Cell Symposium, June 24th, 2010. Gynecol Oncol. 2011;121:407–15.
23. DeLair D, Oliva E, Köbel M, Macias A, Gilks CB, Soslow RA. Morphologic spectrum of immunohistochemically characterized clear cell carcinoma of the ovary: a study of 155 cases. Am J Surg Pathol. 2011;35:36–44.
24. Jones S, Wang TL, Shih IM, Mao TL, Nakayama K, Roden R, Glas R, Slamon D, Diaz Jr LA, Vogelstein B, Kinzler KW, Velculescu VE, Papadopoulos N. Frequent mutations of chromatin remodeling gene ARID1A in ovarian clear cell carcinoma. Science. 2010;330:228–31.
25. Wiegand KC, Shah SP, Al-Agha OM, Zhao Y, Tse K, Zeng T, Senz J, McConechy MK, Anglesio MS, Kalloger SE, Yang W, Heravi-Moussavi A, Giuliany R, Chow C, Fee J, Zayed A, Prentice L, Melnyk N, Turashvili G, Delaney AD, Madore J, Yip S, McPherson AW, Ha G, Bell L, Fereday S, Tam A, Galletta L, Tonin PN, Provencher D, Miller D, Jones SJ, Moore RA, Morin GB, Oloumi A, Boyd N, Aparicio SA, Shih IM, Mes-Masson AM, Bowtell DD, Hirst M, Gilks B, Marra MA, Huntsman DG. ARID1A mutations in endometriosis-associated ovarian carcinomas. N Engl J Med. 2010;363:1532–43.
26. Yamamoto S, Tsuda H, Takano M, Tamai S, Matsubara O. Loss of ARID1A protein expression occurs as an early event in ovarian clear-cell carcinoma development and frequently coexists with PIK3CA mutations. Mod Pathol. 2012;25:615–24.
27. Yamamoto S, Tsuda H, Miyai K, Takano M, Tamai S, Matsubara O. Gene amplification and protein overexpression of MET are common events in ovarian clear-cell adenocarcinoma: their roles in tumor progression and prognostication of the patient. Mod Pathol. 2011;24:1146–55.
28. Austin RM, Norris HJ. Malignant Brenner tumor and transitional cell carcinoma of the ovary: a comparison. Int J Gynecol Pathol. 1987;6:29–39.
29. Mano MS, Rosa DD, Azambuja E, Ismael G, Braga S, D'Hondt V, Piccart M, Awada A. Current management of ovarian carcinosarcoma. Int J Gynecol Cancer. 2007;17:316–24.
30. Pins MR, Young RH, Daly WJ, Scully RE. Primary squamous cell carcinoma of the ovary. Report of 37 cases. Am J Surg Pathol. 1996;20:823–33.

31. Prat J, Scully RE. Cellular fibromas and fibrosarcomas of the ovary: a comparative clinico-pathologic analysis of seventeen cases. Cancer. 1981;47:2663–70.

32. Irving JA, Alkushi A, Young RH, Clement PB. Cellular fibromas of the ovary: a study of 75 cases including 40 mitotically active tumors emphasizing their distinction from fibrosarcoma. Am J Surg Pathol. 2006;30:929–38.

33. Shah SP, Köbel M, Senz J, Morin RD, Clarke BA, Wiegand KC, Leung G, Zayed A, Mehl E, Kalloger SE, Sun M, Giuliany R, Yorida E, Jones S, Varhol R, Swenerton KD, Miller D, Clement PB, Crane C, Madore J, Provencher D, Leung P, DeFazio A, Khattra J, Turashvili G, Zhao Y, Zeng T, Glover JN, Vanderhyden B, Zhao C, Parkinson CA, Jimenez-Linan M, Bowtell DD, Mes-Masson AM, Brenton JD, Aparicio SA, Boyd N, Hirst M, Gilks CB, Marra M, Huntsman DG. Mutation of FOXL2 in granulosa-cell tumors of the ovary. N Engl J Med. 2009;360:2719–29.

34. Miller K, McCluggage WG. Prognostic factors in ovarian adult granulosa cell tumour. J Clin Pathol. 2008;61:881–4.

Care of the Elderly Ovarian Cancer Patient: The Surgical Challenge

4

Kathleen Moore

Contents

Introduction

The elderly population, typically defined as greater than 65 years of age, is the most rapidly growing age bracket in the United States. The US Census estimates that by the year 2020, there will be over 54 million people living in the United States over the age of 65 (13.5 %) and by 2040, this will increase to over 80 million people (20.4 %) [34]. In 2020, approximately 2 % of people will be greater than 80 years of age, and this percentage will double by 2050 [34].

K. Moore, MD
Gynecologic Oncology, The Stephenson Cancer Center, University of Oklahoma,
Norman, OK, USA
e-mail: Kathleen.Moore@ouhsc.edu

© Springer International Publishing Switzerland 2016
G. Freyer (ed.), *Ovarian Cancer in Elderly Patients*,
DOI 10.1007/978-3-319-23588-2_4

Cancer is recognized as a disease of the elderly with over 50 % of new cases being diagnosed after age 65 and over 70 % of deaths from cancer occurring in this same age group [41, 42]. Ovarian cancer, predominantly a disease of postmenopausal women, should also increase in prevalence with an increasingly aged population. In the United States in 2013, there will be over 22,240 new cases and over 14,030 deaths [3]. According to SEER data, 54 % of cases occur in women less than 64 years of age; 20.1 % between 65 and 74; 17.6 % between 75 and 84 and 8.1 % > 85 years [14]. With increasing age, there is an increased prevalence of comorbid conditions, polypharmacy, functional dependence, cognitive impairment, depression, frailty, poor nutrition, and limited social support [9]. Given these many potential limitations, it is not surprising that many elderly patients who present with advanced ovarian cancer receive less aggressive therapies than their younger counterparts and have poorer disease-specific outcomes.

A proportion of patients, both aged and not, present with advanced ovarian malignancies for whom primary cytoreductive surgery (CRS) is not indicated – for example – those with very poor performance status and those with obvious unresectable disease. For the remainder of patients who present, including those >70 and >80 year of age, the ability to assess who is fit enough to undergo aggressive CRS followed by chemotherapy and who should be offered an alternative pathway such as neoadjuvant chemotherapy (NACT) and interval cytoreductive surgery (iCRS) or primary chemotherapy alone – is an unmet need. Ovarian cancer patients have unique presentations and challenges as compared to other solid tumors. For example, CRS for ovarian cancer requires a large abdominal laparotomy; even in the face of widespread malignancy, an aggressive surgery is performed which may include bowel resections, splenectomy, and other procedures as compared to most other solid tumors where widespread malignancy is considered a contraindication to CRS. Patients may present with poor nutrition values and poor performance status due to rapid accumulation of ascites and not due to underlying medical comorbidities. If we use a generalized preoperative assessment for these patients, we may exclude many who might benefit from aggressive primary CRS. However, by not validating a preoperative tool in this vulnerable population, we risk excess morbidity and mortality in those patients with too little reserve to tolerate primary CRS followed by chemotherapy.

The Role of Surgical Debulking

The practice of performing primary CRS followed by platinum-based chemotherapy versus NACT with iCRS surgery is a controversial topic internationally. The survival benefit of performing a primary CRS has never been proven in prospective trials, but ancillary data analysis of several cooperative group chemotherapy trials found that residual tumor <1 cm was associated with superior survival as compared to patients with residual disease >1 cm [39]. This goal has shifted further to obtaining no gross residual (NGR) disease at the conclusion of CRS. In fact, studies suggest that those patients whose surgeons can achieve zero residual tumor at time of

CRS have significantly longer survival than those patients previously considered optimal at 0–1 cm [21]. Gynecologic Oncology Group (GOG) protocol 158 compared paclitaxel/cisplatin to paclitaxel/carboplatin in patients with < 1 cm residual disease following surgery and found median progression free survival (PFS) of 19–20 months and overall survival (OS) of 49–57 months [27]. GOG 183 compared a variety of doublets and triplets versus paclitaxel/carboplatin and separated out no gross residual from gross residual < 1 cm. Patients with gross residual < 1 cm had median PFS and OS of 16 and 40 months. Those with no gross residual had median PFS and OS of 29 and 68 months [31]. Two ancillary data analyses have been performed of cooperative group clinical trial data from the GOG as well as AGO-OVAR. These studies both included clinical trial data from primary platinum-based chemotherapy trials (stage III/IV GOG and stage II-IV AGO-OVAR) administered following primary CRS. Ancillary analysis of GOG, primary platinum-based intravenous chemotherapy regimens, reported a median OS of 71.9 months for those patients with NGR, 42.4 months for those patients with gross disease < 1 cm and 35 months for those patients with residual disease >1 cm [37]. A similar analysis of AGO-OVAR cooperative group trials reported median OS of 99.1, 36.2 and 29.6 months, respectively [11]. Change et al. published a meta-analysis evaluating the effect of residual disease on survival across cooperative group trials and other well-designed trials and reported median OS 77.8, 39 and 31.1 months, respectively[7].

An ancillary review of GOG protocols 114 and 172, both intraperitoneal delivery of cisplatin following primary CRS, found median PFS and OS of 43 and 110 months among those patients who started chemotherapy with NGR disease [19].

An alternative to primary CRS is NACT followed by iCRS. This has been evaluated in two large prospective randomized trials comparing primary CRS to NACT and iCRS. Both these trials (EORTC 55971 and CHORUS) enrolled patients with large volume disease consistent with FIGO stage III/IV disease. Vergote et al. reporting for EORTC 55971 found PFS and OS were identical in the two arms (12 months and 30 months, respectively), but perioperative complications were lower in those patients receiving neoadjuvant chemotherapy. Of note, however, the strongest predictor of survival was CRS to no gross residual disease and the authors note that careful analysis of important predictive factors of debulking surgery resulting in no residual tumor, such as comorbidities, age, disease burden, location of metastatic sites, performance status, and stage should be taken into account when deciding on NACT or primary CRS [36]. Also of interest is there was no effect of age > or < 70 on benefit or harm of either surgical approach in terms of effect on OS [36]. The CHORUS trial has only been presented in abstract form thus far but found very consistent results in that there was no demonstrated benefit for pCRS over iCRS in terms of survival with median PFS of 10.3 and 11.7 months and median OS of 22.8 and 24.5 months, respectively [15].

Although these two well-designed prospective trials failed to demonstrate a difference in survival based on timing of surgical cytoreduction, there are questions regarding patient selection and the comparatively low survival outcomes when compared to primary chemotherapy data following pCRS as outlined above (Table 4.1).

Table 4.1 Comparison of outcomes across prospective trials of chemotherapy following pCRS and trials of timing of surgical cytoreduction

	AGO-OVAR [11]	GOG [37]	EORTC 55971 pCRS iCRS [36]	CHORUS pCRS iCRS [15]
Suboptimal > 1 cm	29.6 months	35.0 months	26 months 25	22.8–24.5
Gross optimal ≤ 1 cm	36.2 months	42.4 months	32 months 27	
NGR	99 months	71.9 months	45 months 38	
Age	58.9	57	62–63	65–66
PS	0 38 %	0 41 %	0 45 %	0 13 %
	2 10.4 %	2 8.5 %	2–3 32 %	2–3 20 %
Stage	II 8.9 %	III 100 %	IIIc 76.5–	III 75 %
	III 74 %		75.7 %	IV 25 %
	IV 17 %		IV 22.9–24.3 %	

While there does appear to be a significant survival benefit in achieving no gross residual tumor and proceeding with platinum-based chemotherapy, this table is a good reminder of how cross study comparisons can be misleading. If one looks at the patient criteria, we see that both EORTC 55971 and CHORUS had patients whose median age was about a decade older than either the GOG or AGO-OVAR studies, had significantly more patients with performance status 2, and had significantly more patients with stage IV disease.

These studies have provided important guidance as to identifying patients who would be better served with NACT and iCRS versus pCRS, and this group undoubtedly includes some elderly patients; however, we are still faced with uncertainty regarding the best sequence of therapies for those patients felt medically fit enough to undergo pCRS and attempt to maximize survival. A proportion of elderly patients will fall into this category as well.

Outcomes Among Elderly Patients Who Undergo CRS: What Do We Know?

As discussed above, the goal of CRS, whether it be pCRS or iCRS is to achieve NGR. This outcome is achieved in a variable proportion of patients dependent on presenting disease burden and surgeon skill and comes at a significant cost in terms of morbidity and mortality. Many single institution studies have been published exploring this issue in the "elderly patient" with a variety of definitions of elderly and a variety of outcomes – pointing to the dearth of prospective data in the area (Table 4.2).

Because of the retrospective nature of these works and the variety in endpoints studied, it is difficult to summarize outcomes for anything other than postoperative death which seems to increase markedly with age. If we classify elderly as > 65, prevalence of postoperative death is 0–10.3 % (with 0 % in the series with almost 50 % of patients undergoing iCRS) [12, 20, 23]. If we change the cutpoint for

Table 4.2 Published case series of outcomes and survival with elderly ovary cancer

Author	Age	No of pts	PFS (mo)	OS	Postoperative mortality	Postoperative complications	Primary surgery	NACT selected
Marchetti [23]	≥65 years	29	NA	19.2 months	3 (10.3 %)	NA	28 (96.6 %)	1 (3.4 %)
Susini [32]	≥70 years	51	NA	NA	NA	NA	51 (100 %)	Study exclusion
Cloven [10]	≥80 years	18	NA	6 months	2 (11.1 %)	– Cardiac: 7 (39 %) – Sepsis: 3 (16.7 %) – Pneumonia: 1 (5.6 %)	16 (88.9 %)	3 (16.7 %)
Bruchim [6]	≥70 years	46	NA	NA	2 (4.3 %)	NA	25 (54.3 %)	13 (43.3 %)
Wright [38]	≥70 years	46	NA	NA	0	– ICU admission: 20 % – Infection: 8 % – Delirium: 5 % – Wound: 3 % – Ileus: 2 % – Arrhythmia: 2 % – VTE: 1 %	46 (100 %)	Study exclusion
Uyar [35]	≥70 years	131	NA	70–79 years: 52 months ≥80 years: 36 months p = .07	NA	– Overall: 23 %	105 (80 %)	26 (20 %)
Alphs [2]	≥75 years	78	NA	19 months	7 (9 %)	– Wound infection: 13 (16.7 %) – Ileus: 5 (6.4 %)	78 (100 %)	Study exclusion
Moore [25]	≥80 years	85	NA	1°surgery: 2 years survival 51 % 1°chemo: 2 years survival 27 %	9 (13 %)	– Cardiac: 17 % – Pulmonary: 26 % – GI: 22 % – Heme/infectious: 62 % – Mental status: 10 % – Surgical site: 23 %	68 (80 %)	17 (20 %)

(continued)

Table 4.2 (continued)

Author	Age	No of pts	PFS (mo)	OS	Postoperative mortality	Postoperative complications	Primary surgery	NACT selected
Moore [26]	≥80 years	39	NA	NA	NA	NA	39 (100 %)	Study exclusion
McLean [24]	≥80 years	34	NA	24	0	– Ileus: 29.4 % – Pneumonia: 6.1 % – Wound infection: 3.1 % – Sepsis: 3 %	27 (79.4 %)	7 (20.6 %)
Chereau [8]	≥70 years	29	2 years: 35 % 5 years: 23 %	5 years: 55 %	1 (3.4 %)	– Overall: 3 (10 %) – Infection: 2 (7 %) – Febrile morbidity: 1 (3 %) – Pleural effusion: 1 (3 %)	29 (100 %)	Study exclusion
Langstraat [21]	≥65 years	280	NA	NA	12 (4.3 %)	Overall: 32 (11.4 %)	280 (100 %)	Study exclusion
Fanfani [12]	≥65 years	164	65–74 years: 12 months ≥75 years: 21 months	NA	0	Overall: 65–74 years: 11 (11.2 %) ≥75 years: 8 (25 %)	75 (45.7 %)	89 (54.3 %)

No number, *PFS* progression free survival, *OS* overall survival, *NACT* neoadjuvant chemotherapy, *NA* not applicable, recorded, or extractable from the publication for this specific subset of patients, 1 primary elderly to >70, the range is 0–9 % [2, 6, 8, 32, 35, 38]. Finally, if we set the cutpoint at age >80, postoperative death is reported in 0–13 % of series [10, 24, 25].

In order to make the more informed decisions regarding how to care of elderly patients with ovarian cancer and provide them with the most accurate counseling, we need good estimates of the following 4 outcomes: (1) postoperative death, (2) postoperative morbidity, (3) non-traditional discharge, and (4) deviations from or elimination of planned chemotherapy.

Postoperative Death

Among the possible complications following CRS, postoperative death is the most significant. Case series report prevalence of 0–13 % with significant variability in populations. Thrall et al. published a SEER-Medicare evaluation which sought to identify the prevalence of 30-day postoperative mortality among patients undergoing CRS and develop a predictive nomogram for this complication. This study contained only women >65 years and included those undergoing both pCRS and iCRS. They found an overall 30-day postoperative mortality rate of 8.22 %. However, when patients who were admitted and underwent surgery emergently were evaluated separately, the rate of 5.56 % among scheduled and 20.12 % among emergent cases. Age was highly associated with postoperative death in both these groups. When evaluated as a continuous variable among patients admitted for scheduled surgery, each year over age 65 was associated with a 7.5 % increase in the risk of 30-day mortality (95 % CI 1.06–1.10). Among patients admitted and operated on emergently, each year over age 65 was associated with a 2.8 % increase in the risk of 30-day mortality (95 % CI 1.01–1.05).

Among those patients admitted for elective surgery who had a history of NACT, the 30-day mortality was 70 % lower than those who underwent pCRS (1.82 vs. 6.13 %).

When evaluating patients admitted for elective surgery with no history of NACT, the risk of 30-day mortality could be divided into low (<5 %), intermediate (5–10 %), and high (>10 %) risk based on age, stage, and comorbidity score. The highest risk group included patients 75 years of age or older, with stage IV disease or stage III disease plus a comorbidity score of 1 or more. This group comprised 25.7 % of the patients and had a 30-day postoperative mortality of 12.7 % which accounted for 50 % of the deaths in the entire cohort [33].

This risk score has not been validated in prospective trial but is valuable information for evaluating patients and making treatment decisions based on the best information available.

Postoperative Morbidity

Postoperative complications are important to avoid, not only for the obvious reason of eliminating patient discomfort and risk but also because certain complications are associated in a reduction in overall survival. This is not to say that patients die of their complications, which would be postoperative death, but the complication compromises the ability of the patient to survive their cancer. National Surgical

Table 4.3 Postoperative complications by age and radical procedures [39]

	<50 6654 (23 %)	50–59 7226 (25.2 %)	60–69 6903 (24.1 %)	70–79 5660 (19.8 %)	>80 2208 (7.7 %)	P value
Any complication	1138 (17.1 %)	1461 (20.2 %)	1763 (25.5 %)	1680 (29.7 %)	696 (31.5 %)	<0.0001
Surgical site	365 (5.5 %)	458 (6.3 %)	566 (8.2 %)	508 (9 %)	235 (10.6 %)	<0.0001
Medical complication	734 (11 %)	992 (13.7 %)	1169 (16.9 %)	1171 (20.7 %)	470 (21.3 %)	<0.0001
Infectious	207 (3.1 %)	290 (4.0 %)	402 (5.8 %)	435 (7.7 %)	189 (8.6 %)	<0.0001
	% (OR)	% (OR)	% (OR)	% (OR)	% (OR)	
0 radical procedure	10.2 (ref)	12.2 (ref)	15.6 (ref)	18.5 (ref)	18.3 (ref)	
1 radical procedure	15.7 (1.28)	18.4 (1.35)	20.2 (1.21)	24.9 (1.29)	28.9 (17)	<0.05
≥2 radical procedure	23.7 (2.06)	29.7 (2.37)	25.7 (1.62)	33.1 (1.82)	33.3 (2.0)	<0.05

Quality Improvement Program (NSQIP) data found that the most important determinant of decreased survival following surgery for patients with solid tumors with occurrence of a major complication [16]. These data exist in ovary cancer as well where the occurrence of 2 or more complications increased the risk of death from cancer (HR 1.31 95 % CI 1.15–1.49) [40]. Wright et al., evaluating the Nationwide Inpatient Sample registry of patients admitted for ovarian cancer surgery, found that perioperative complications increased with age. This study could not separate patients who underwent pCRS and those who underwent iCRS and so they are presented together. Among the 28,651 patients included, those patients <50 years of age had a 17.1 % complication rate as compared to 29.7 % in patients aged 70–79 and 31.5 % in patients >80. These trends held regardless of categorization as a medical, surgical, or infectious complication. Not surprisingly, rates of complications also increased by age and by the number of radical procedures performed at the time of surgery. Patients over 70 who required 2 or more radical procedures (bowel resections, diaphragm resections, etc) at the time of surgery had complications in 33 % of cases. One radical procedure in the age range resulted in 25 % with major complications. Given the commonality of radical procedures during pCRS to achieve NGR, these are useful estimates in counseling patients and determining the best sequence of therapy [39] (Table 4.3).

Non-traditional Discharge (NTD)

Data on discharge to nursing home or rehabilitation facility are difficult to obtain retrospectively. Again using NIS data, Wright et al. characterized NTD by age and by number of radical procedures. Overall, NTD increases with age from 1 % only 1.0 % of patients <50 compared to 14.0 % of patients age 70–79 and 33.3 % of patients >80. When the number of radical procedures is factored in, patients age 70–79 with one radical procedure have NTD in 12 % of cases vs. 30 % in patients >80. For 2 radical procedures the rates are 17 and 40 %, respectively, and if one performs greater than 2 radical procedures the rates are 25 and 49 %, respectively [39]. Among elderly patients who are independent, maintenance of their independence and avoidance of institutionalization may be of higher priority than the possibility of superior overall survival. Preoperative counseling for this possibility and integration into treatment decisions are essential.

Effect on Chemotherapy Delivery

There are three potential issues with chemotherapy delivery as related to postoperative complications: (1) omission of chemotherapy altogether, (2) substantial delay in initiation of chemotherapy, and (3) significant modification in planned chemotherapy. The latter two issues are difficult if not impossible to classify from retrospective studies because there is rarely documentation of what chemotherapy and doses (or route of administration) was planned, and reasons for delay in chemotherapy vary widely across practice patterns, patient decisions, and postoperative complications causing delay. Omission of chemotherapy is easier to identify following surgery. SEER data report 12 % of patients fail to ever initiate chemotherapy, but that this is not related to complications or number of radical procedures. Instead it was related to age, single marital status, stage, mucinous histology, and multiple comorbidities ($p < 0.05$). In this study, delay did not appear to effect outcomes until >12 weeks delay which occurred in 8 % of patients >80 as compared to 4.2 % overall [40]. Aletti et al. reported data from 3 academic institutions and found a rate of 4.7–8.2 % failure to initiate chemotherapy, and this failure was related to ASA grade and surgical complexity score (<0.001 and $p = 0.003$) [1]. In EORTC 55971, 22/336 (6.6 %) patients did not receive chemotherapy following pCRS. Most of these patients did not receive therapy because of excessive postsurgery complications or the diagnosis of another primary tumor. Median survival for these patients was 2.7 months [36 – supplemental appendix].

In summary, the timing of CRS remains controversial with an abundance of ancillary and retrospective data demonstrating superiority of pCRS to NGD and recent prospective trials demonstrating no benefit to pCRS or iCRS – at least in large volume stage IIIC and IV disease. The higher incidence of complications in pCRS vs. iCRS is not controversial, and the increasing rate with age and comorbidities is clear as well. The critical age cutpoints for key complications appears to be age 75 for postoperative mortality, age 70 for postoperative morbidity and NTD, and age 80 for omission of chemotherapy. The anticipated benefits in survival achieved by pCRS to NGR must be balanced with the perceived tolerance of anticipated complications and the effect those complications may have on patient survival as well.

Models of Preoperative Assessment

Currently there is no widely accepted, validated preoperative assessment to help triage patients to pCRS or iCRS. This decision is based on the surgeon's appraisal of their fitness to undergo radical surgery and lacks objective measures. Traditional models of preoperative assessment, including Lee, Eagle, ASA, and others, do not take into account the multisystem assessment needed to evaluate ovarian cancer patients. Exploration of other preoperative assessments is ongoing to include assessments of frailty, the comprehensive geriatrics assessment, and the preoperative assessment of cancer in the elderly (PACE).

Frailty

Frailty is defined as a state of decreased physiologic reserve and increased susceptibility to suffer disability in response to stressors [22, 29]. How frailty is measured varies between a physical assessment and a more physiologic assessment.

Makary et al. used a validated scoring system of physical frailty in a prospective study of patients >65 years of age presenting for elective surgery. The frailty score was based on five domains, which included weight loss, weakness, exhaustion, low physical activity, and slowed walking speed [5, 13, 22].

This frailty score was then compared to more conventional preoperative assessments such as the ASA score, Lee's revised cardiac index, and Eagle score. Of 594 patients, 62 (10.4 %) were frail and 186 (31.3 %) were intermediately frail. Frailty was found to correlate with postoperative complications with an adjusted odds ratio of 1.78–2.13 for intermediately frail patients and 2.48–3.15 in frail patients. Frailty was also correlated with increased length of stay (65–89 % longer stays for frail patients) as well as non-traditional discharge [22].

Other investigators have looked at physiologic frailty as a predictor of outcome in preoperative patients. Domains studied included comorbidity, function, nutrition, cognition, geriatric syndrome assessment, and extrinsic frailty (social support) [29].

Using this assessment of frailty for 110 patients ≥65 undergoing elective surgery with planned ICU admission found that the following factors were associated most closely with 6-month mortality: cognitive dysfunction, lower albumin, having fallen in the past 6 months, lower hematocrit, functional dependence, and increased comorbidities. Having four or more of these markers predicted 6-month mortality with a sensitivity of 86 % [30]. In a follow-up study with 223 patients and using the same assessments, the authors found that timed up and go >15 s, any functional dependence, Charlson score ≥3, and hematocrit ≤35 were the variables most predictive of postoperative institutionalization [30].

Comprehensive Geriatric Assessment (CGA)

The CGA is a multidisciplinary assessment of the elderly patient across multiple domains including functional status (activities of daily living (ADL), independent activities of daily living (IADL), and gait speed), history of geriatric syndromes (falls/imbalance), cognition, mood disorders, comorbidities, and social support. The CGA has been adapted for use in elderly cancer patients to try and predict complications due to chemotherapy and make appropriate modifications for those patients at risk [28]. Studies evaluating the CGA in the preoperative setting are rare to date with two notable exceptions. Kristjansoon et al. published and evaluated the CGA in patients undergoing surgery for colorectal cancer. They classified patients as fit, intermediate, or frail and found that those patients classified as intermediate or frail were more likely to have postoperative complications than those classified as fit [18]. Using an abbreviated assessment, Kothari et al. used the CGA to predict postoperative outcomes in patients undergoing thoracic surgery and found that answers to certain questions predicted postoperative morbidity [17].

Preoperative Assessment of Cancer in the Elderly (PACE)

The PACE tool was developed to combine elements of the CGA with surgical risk assessment tools. Instruments included in the PACE are a mini-mental state inventory, ADLs, IADLs, GDS, brief fatigue inventory (BFI), ECOG performance status (PS), ASA, and Satariano's index of comorbidities. This tool has been studied prospectively among 460 patients undergoing surgery for breast cancer, gastrointestinal cancer, genitourinary cancer, and others. Endpoints of interest were 30-day morbidity, mortality, and hospital stay. They found no significant association of age with postoperative complications. IADL, moderate to severe BFI, and abnormal PS were most predictive of 30-day morbidity. ADL, IADL, and PS were associated with extended hospital stay. There were too few deaths at 30 days to draw conclusions [4, 27]. While promising, use of the PACE in a population of patients with "higher risk surgeries" has not yet been performed.

Given the importance of the issue of preoperative assessment in general as well as the increasing geriatric population, a position paper was released in 2012 outlining best practices for optimal preoperative assessment of the geriatric patient [9]. In this document, the authors provide a checklist which covers the expected surgical assessment. This is a comprehensive assessment which incorporates almost all domains described in the assessment tools above.

Conclusions

There is no validated intrument for assessing of the elderly or performance status challenged ovarian cancer patient does not yet exist. There are several excellent assessments under study for breast and other solid tumor which may lend themselves to this unique population, but prospective study is imperative to remove the guess work from assessing a patient's fitness for surgery.

References

1. Aletti GD, et al. A new frontier for quality of care in gynecologic oncology surgery: multi-institutional assessment of shortterm outcomes for ovarian cancer using a risk-adjusted model. Gynecol Oncol. 2007;107(1):99–106. Epub 2007 Jun 28.

2. Alphs HH, et al. Predictors of surgical outcome and survival among elderly women diagnosed with ovarian and primary peritoneal cancer. Gynecol Oncol. 2006;103:1048–53. American Cancer Society. Cancer Facts & Figures 2013. Atlanta: American Cancer Society 2013.
3. American Cancer Society. Cancer facts & figures 2013. Atlanta: American Cancer Society; 2013.
4. Audisio RA, et al. Shall we operate? Preoperative assessment in elderly cancer patients (PACE) can help. A SIOG surgical task force prospective study. Crit Rev Oncol Hematol. 2008;65(2): 156–63.
5. Bandeen-Roche K, et al. Phenotype of frailty: characterization in the women's health and aging studies. J Gerontol A Boil Sci Med Sci. 2006;61:262–6.
6. Bruchim I, et al. Age contrasts in clinical characteristics and pattern of care in patients with epithelial ovarian cancer. Gynecol Oncol. 2002;86:274–8.
7. Chang SJ, et al. Prognostic significance of systematic lymphadenectomy as part of primary debulking surgery in patients with advanced ovarian cancer. Gynecol Oncol. 2012;126(3): 381–6. doi: 10.1016/j.ygyno.2012.05.014. Epub 2012 May 18.
8. Chereau E, et al. Ovarian cancer in the elderly: impact of surgery on morbidity and survival. Eur J Surg Oncol. 2011;37:537–42.
9. Chow WB, et al. Optimal preoperative assessment of the geriatric surgical patient: a best practices guideline from the American College of Surgeon National Surgical Quality Improvement Program and the American Geriatrics Society. J Am Coll Surg. 2012;215:453–66.
10. Cloven NG, et al. Management of ovarian cancer in patients older than 80 years of age. Gynecol Oncol. 1999;73:137–9.
11. Du Bois A, et al. Role of surgical outcome as prognostic factor in advanced epithelial ovarian cancer: a combined exploratory analysis of 3 prospectively randomized phase 3 multicenter trials: by the Arbeitsgemeinschaft Gynaekologische Onkologie Studiengruppe Ovarialkarzinom (AGO-OVAR) and the Groupe d'Investigateurs Nationaux Pour les Etudes des Cancers de l'Ovaire (GINECO). Cancer. 2009;115(6):1234–44. doi: 10.1002/cncr.24149.
12. Fanfani F, et al. Elderly and very elderly advanced ovarian cancer patients: does the age influence the surgical management? Eur J Surg Oncol. 2012;38:1204–10.
13. Fried LP, et al. Frailty in older adults: evidence for a phenotype. J Gerontol A Biol Sci Med Sci. 2001;56:M146–56.
14. Howlander N, et al. SEER cancer statistics review, 1975–2009 (Vintage 2009 Populations). Bethesda: National Cancer Institute. http://seer.cancer.gov/csr/1975_2009_pops09/
15. Kehoe S, et al. JCO ASCO annual meeting. Proc Am Soc Clin Oncol. 2013;1354.
16. Khuri SF, et al. Determinants of long-term survival after major surgery and the adverse effect of postoperative complications. Participants in the VA National Surgical Quality Improvement Program. Ann Surg. 2005;242(3):326–41; discussion 341–3.
17. Kothari A, et al. Components of geriatric assessments predict thoracic surgery outcomes. J Surg Res. 2011;166:5–13.
18. Kristjansson SR, et al. Comprehensive geriatric assessment can predict complications in elderly patients after elective surgery for colorectal cancer: a prospective observational cohort study. Crit Rev Oncol Hematol. 2010;76:208–17.
19. Landrum L, et al. Prognostic factors for stage III epithelial ovarian cancer treated with Intraperitoneal chemotherapy: a gynecologic oncology group study. Gynecol Oncol. 2012;125: S3–167 abstract 56.
20. Langstraat C, Cliby WA. Consideration in the surgical management of ovarian cancer in the elderly. Curr Treat Options Oncol. 2013;14(1):12–21 Epub nov 2012.
21. Langstraat C, et al. Morbidity, mortality and overall survival in elderly women undergoing primary surgical debulking for ovarian cancer: a delicate balance requiring individualization. Gynecol Oncol. 2012;123:187–91.
22. Makary MA, et al. Frailty as a predictor of surgical outcomes in older patients. J Am Coll Surg. 2010;210:901–8.
23. Marchetti DL, et al. Treatment of advanced ovarian carcinoma in the elderly. Gynecol Oncol. 1993;49:86–91.

24. McLean KA, et al. Ovarian cancer in the elderly: outcomes with neoadjuvant chemotherapy or primary cytoreduction. Gynecol Oncol. 2010;118:43–6.
25. Moore KN, et al. Ovarian cancer in the octogenarian: does the paradigm of aggressive cytoreductive surgery and chemotherapy still apply? Gynecol Oncol. 2008;110:133–9.
26. Moore KN, et al. Adjuvant chemotherapy for the "oldest old" ovarian cancer patients: can we anticipate toxicity-related treatment failure in a vulnerable population? Cancer. 2009;115: 1472–80.
27. Ozols Pope D, et al. Pre operative assessment of cancer in the elderly (PACE): a comprehensive assessment of underlying characteristics of elderly patients prior to elective surgery. Surg Oncol. 2006;15(4):189–97.
28. Puts MTE, et al. Use of geriatic assessment for older adults in oncology setting: a systematic review. J Natl Cancer Inst. 2012;104:1133–63.
29. Robinson TH, et al. Redefining geriatric preoperative assessment using frailty, disability and co-morbidity. Ann Surg. 2009;250:449–55.
30. Robinson TH, et al. Accumulated frailty characteristics predict post operative discharge institutionalization in the geriatric patient. J Am Coll Surg. 2011;213:37–44.
31. Rodriguez N, et al. Upper abdominal procedures in advanced stage ovarian or primary peritoneal carcinoma patients with minimal or no gross residual disease: an analysis of Gynecologic Oncology Group (GOG) 182. Gynecol Oncol. 2013;130(3):487–92. doi: 10.1016/j.ygyno.2013.06.017. Epub 2013 Jun 17.
32. Susini T, et al. Gynecologic oncologic surgery in the elderly: a retrospective analysis of 213 patients. Gynecol Oncol. 1999;75:437–43.
33. Thrall MM, et al. Thirty day mortality after primary cytoreductive surgery for advanced ovarian cancer in the elderly. Obstet Gynecol. 2011;118(3):537–47.
34. US Census Bureau. US interim projections by age, sex, race and Hispanic origin. 2004. http://www.census.gov/inc/www/usinterim,inj/internet. Release date: 18 Mar 2004.
35. Uyar D, et al. Treatment patterns by decade of life in elderly women (> or =70 years of age) with ovarian cancer. Gynecol Oncol. 2005;98:403–8.
36. Vergote I, et al. Neoadjuvant chemotherapy or primary surgery in stage IIIc or IV ovarian cancer. N Engl J Med. 2010;363:943–53.
37. Winter WE 3rd, et al. Tumor residual after surgical cytoreduction in prediction of clinical outcome in stage IV epithelial ovarian cancer: a Gynecologic Oncology Group Study. J Clin Oncol. 2008;26(1):83–9. Epub 2007 Nov 19.
38. Wright JD, et al. Morbidity of cytoreductive surgery in the elderly. Am J Obstet Gynecol. 2004;190:1398–400.
39. Wright JD, et al. Defining the limits of radical cytoreductive surgery for ovarian cancer. Gynecol Oncol. 2011;123:467–73.
40. Wright JD, et al. Effect of radical cytoreductive surgery on omission and delay of chemotherapy for advanced-stage ovarian cancer. Obstet Gynecol. 2012;120(4):871–81.
41. Yancik R. Population aging and cancer: a cross-national concern. Cancer J. 2005;11:437–41. (25): 3457–3465.
42. Yancik R, Ries LA. Cancer in older persons: an international issue in an aging world. Semin Oncol. 2004;31:128–36.

Chemotherapy: First-Line Strategy

5

Olivia Le Saux, Claire Falandry, and Gilles Freyer

Contents

Introduction

Ovarian cancer (OC) is the seventh most common cancer and the eighth cause of death from cancer in women worldwide [1]. However, there are large variations in its incidence and mortality across the world. The highest incidence areas are to be

O. Le Saux (✉)
Medical Oncology Department, Centre Hospitalier Lyon Sud - Institut de Cancérologie des Hospices Civils de Lyon, 165, Chemin du Grand Revoyet, Pierre-Bénite 69310, France

Lyon 1 University, EMR 3738, Faculté de Médecine Lyon-Sud, 165, Chemin du Petit Revoyet - BP12, Oullins Cedex 69921, France
e-mail: olivia.lesaux@gmail.com

G. Falandry, MD, PhD
Geriatric Oncology Department, Centre Hospitalier Lyon Sud - Institut de Cancérologie des Hospices Civils de Lyon, 165, Chemin du Grand Revoyet, Pierre-Bénite 69310, France

G. Freyer, MD, PhD
HCL Cancer Institute, Medical Oncology, and Université de Lyon, Lyon, France

© Springer International Publishing Switzerland 2016   49
G. Freyer (ed.), *Ovarian Cancer in Elderly Patients*,
DOI 10.1007/978-3-319-23588-2_5

found in Europe and North America where OC is the leading cause of death from gynecological cancer [2]. Therefore, OC is an important public health issue in developed countries.

Incidence and mortality increase with age with incidence peaking between the ages of 75 and 79 and mortality between the ages of 80 and 84. About 50 % of cases are diagnosed in women over 65 [2]. This ratio is expected to increase in the upcoming years as life expectancy improves [3].

Compared with younger patients, OC in elderly patients $\geq$65 years shows some specificity such as [4]:

- A higher and increasing incidence (five times higher than in younger patients),
- Worse prognosis, with a 5-year survival rate of less than 30 % for elderly patients with advanced stage OC (i.e., FIGO stages III–IV) compared to less than 50 % for younger women, with no significant trend in improved survival over time compared to younger patients.

This poor prognosis might be explained by more advanced stages [5] due to delayed diagnosis, by tumor biology [6] or by undertreatment.

In theory, the standard of care for patients with advanced ovarian cancer consists in a surgical and medical strategy (primary maximal debulking surgery and platinum-based chemotherapy). Although some authors consider this strategy as feasible by analogy with the data obtained in younger patients [7], in clinical practice, elderly patients are less likely to undergo surgery and are more likely to have dose reductions, treatment delays, and to be treated with monotherapies [8]. In order to improve the safety profile of this medico-surgical approach, neoadjuvant chemotherapy is gaining interest worldwide in old and frail patients.

Consequently, the purpose of this chapter is to review current evidence regarding first-line chemotherapy for elderly women with advanced epithelial ovarian cancer (EOC). Standard chemotherapy regimen and modified chemotherapy dosing, scheduling, and timing (neoadjuvant or postoperative) will be discussed successively.

Geriatric Assessment

Evaluating functional status, comorbidities, cognition, psychological status, social support, and nutritional status, geriatric assessment (GA) is predictive of chemotherapy toxicity and survival in cancer patients [9, 10] and in ovarian cancer patients [11].

In ovarian cancer, the objective of GA is to assess the patient's fitness for surgery and chemotherapy.

As with preoperative assessment, a test for older patients undergoing chemotherapy is needed. In this respect, the French Groupe d'Investigateurs Nationaux pour l'Etude des Cancers Ovariens (GINECO) has developed a geriatric vulnerability score (GVS) [12]. This tool has been identified among a French cohort of elderly patients $\geq$70 years treated with front-line carboplatin as a single agent. GVS (Table

Table 5.1 Geriatric vulnerability score

Albuminemia	<35 g/L
Lymphopenia	<1 G/L
ADL score	<6
IADL score	<25
HADS score	>14

The number of points is the sum of "yes"

A vulnerable patient is defined as a patient with a GVS ≥3

ADL *Activities of Daily Living*, IADL *Instrumental Activities of Daily Living*, HADS *Hospital Anxiety Depression Scale*

5.1) takes into account five prognostic factors: albuminemia <35 g/l, Activities of Daily Living (ADL) score <6, Instrumental Activities of Daily Living (IADL) score <25, lymphopenia <1 G/l, and Hospital Anxiety Depression Scale (HADS) score >14. With a cutoff ≥3, GVS discriminated two groups with significantly different overall survival (OS), treatment completion rates, severe adverse events rates, and unplanned hospital admission rates.

First-Line Chemotherapy

Background

OC is a relatively chemosensitive tumor in first-line setting. The current standard of first-line chemotherapy in advanced OC has evolved in the recent years from cyclophosphamide-based regimens to the combination of carboplatin AUC 5 and paclitaxel 175 mg/m^2 [13–17].

In elderly patients, as in younger patients, chemotherapy has a strong impact on OS. According to the Surveillance, Epidemiology, and End Results (SEER)-Medicare database, survival improved by 38 % in treated elderly women, a rate similar to the benefits described in randomized controlled trials among younger patients [18]. Yet, only about half of the patients were treated with platinum-based chemotherapy [18]. This supposed undertreatment has also been reported in other retrospective cohorts of elderly patients not receiving any chemotherapy in 17–29 % of cases [19, 20].

Factors associated with decreased prescription of chemotherapy are age independently of comorbidities [21], and comorbidities [22].

Physicians often tend to reduce doses or prescribe partial courses of chemotherapy because older patients are more vulnerable to chemotherapy toxicities [23], particularly cytopenias and neuropathy [24]. As a consequence, dose intensity is not maintained and prognosis tends to worsen.

The most appropriate choice of agents is, as for their younger counterparts, a platinum-taxane doublet [7]. For older patients, several strategies have been evaluated to improve feasibility and tolerability while maintaining dose intensity. They are single-agent therapy with carboplatin, weekly schedules, and different chemotherapy timing (neoadjuvant chemotherapy).

Choice of Agents

Some authors consider that **standard 3-weekly platinum/paclitaxel** regimen is feasible in elderly patients [25]. Results from the Arbeitsgemeinschaft Gynaekologische Onkologie Ovarian Cancer Study Group 3 (AGO-OVAR-3) phase III trial [14] evaluating cisplatin/paclitaxel versus carboplatin/paclitaxel were retrospectively analyzed according to feasibility, toxicity, and quality of life in patients aged ≥70 years. Thirteen percent of enrolled patients in this trial were ≥70 years. Elderly patients received 98 %, 100 %, and 96 % of the recommended paclitaxel, carboplatin, and cisplatin dose, respectively, per cycle even though early discontinuation was more frequent in elderly patients. Quality of life and nonhematological and hematological toxicity were comparable between elderly and younger patients, except for febrile neutropenia (5 % versus <1 %, $p=0.005$). In this older cohort, platinum/paclitaxel appeared to be feasible and tolerable. However, this population, treated under clinical trial conditions, was highly selected, and the results from this age-specific analysis basically give information about "fit" elderly patients.

Nonetheless, in routine practice, elderly patients are extremely heterogeneous [26]: some will tolerate chemotherapy as well as younger women ("fit patients"), while others will experience unpredictable and severe toxicity ("vulnerable patients"). To overcome this variability and therefore to identify patients at risk of severe toxicity, the French Groupe d'Investigateurs Nationaux pour l'Etude des Cancers Ovariens (GINECO) developed a program named "FAG" for "Femme ÂGée" (elderly woman in English) to assess tolerability and feasibility of standard front-line chemotherapy regimens enrolling unselected elderly patients (regardless of initial performance status and surgery status) while identifying geriatric parameters of interest.

The results of three age-specific prospective trials were successively reported:

1. FAG-1 enrolled 83 advanced ovarian carcinoma patients ≥70 years old from July 1998 to October 2000 [11]. Patients received **carboplatin AUC 5 and cyclophosphamide 600 mg/m2, on day 1 of six 28-day cycles**. Median age was 76 years, optimal initial surgery was carried out in 21 % of cases, and performance status (PS) was ≥2 in 44 % of cases. Sixty patients (72 %) received six chemotherapy cycles without severe toxicity (STox) or tumor progression. Multivariate analysis retained three factors as independent predictors of STox: symptoms of depression at baseline ($p=0.006$), dependence ($p=0.048$), and PS ≥ 2 ($p=0.026$). Independent prognostic factors identified for overall survival were depression ($p=0.003$), FIGO stage IV ($p=0.007$), and more than six different comedications per day ($p=0.043$).
2. FAG-2 enrolled 75 patients ≥70 years from September 2001 to April 2004 [27]. Patients received **carboplatin AUC (Area Under the Curve)=5 mg.min/ml and paclitaxel 175 mg/m2administered each 3-week cycle** for six cycles. 68.1 % of the patients completed six courses.

The data of the two studies ($n=155$ patients) were pooled in a retrospective multivariate analysis [27]. Patients in the second study appeared to be in better shape with younger age and lower PS. Independent prognostic factors of poorer OS were the following: increasing age ($p = 0.013$), depression symptoms at baseline ($p < 0.001$), International Federation of Gynecology and Obstetrics stage IV ($p = 0.001$), and use of paclitaxel ($p = 0.025$).

3. FAG-3 enrolled 111 patients ≥70 years from August 2007 to January 2010 [28]. Patients received **carboplatin AUC (Area Under the Curve) = 5 mg.min/ml every 3 weeks** for up to six cycles. The population in this study had a poorer prognostic factor profile on the basis of geriatric and oncologic parameters compared to the two former trials. Median age was 79 years with 41 % of patients aged ≥80 years. PS was ≥2 in 47 % of cases. The median OS was 17.4 months. On the whole, 74 % of patients completed the six-planned chemotherapy cycles [12].

   Many oncologists consider single-agent carboplatin as a safe and effective regimen for the oldest old or frail patients. This consideration is supported by the results of the International Collaboration on Ovarian Neoplasms (ICON) 3 trial reporting no clear evidence that paclitaxel plus carboplatin is more or less effective than carboplatin or CAP (cyclophosphamide, doxorubicin, and cisplatin) in patients >65 years [29].

Weekly dosing of paclitaxel and carboplatin has been evaluated in the phase II Multicenter Italian Trial in Ovarian cancer (MITO-5) study [30]. Eligible patients were ≥70 years but should have a PS ≤2. Patients received carboplatin (AUC 2) + paclitaxel (60 mg/m^2) on days 1, 8, and 15 every 4 weeks, up to six cycles. Twenty-six patients were analyzed (median age 77 years, range 70–84). Fourteen patients had ≥2 comorbidities; 8 and 18 patients had some dependency in ADL or IADL, respectively. Twenty-three patients (88.5 %) were treated without suffering unacceptable toxicity. Median estimated progression-free survival was 13.6 months and median overall survival was 32.0 months. Similarly, the recent phase III MITO-7 trial's results [31], which compared a weekly regimen to the standard 3-weekly regimen, showed similar progression-free survival (PFS) (18.3 versus 17.3 months, respectively) with less cytopenias, less neurotoxicity, and better quality of life scores. Even though age ≥70 showed no significant effect on PFS, PFS benefit with the weekly regimen was more important within the older-age-specific subgroup (HR: 0.70 [0.46–1.07]) (Table 5.2).

Von Gruenigen et al. recently presented preliminary results of an elderly-specific prospective trial to study chemotherapy toxicity on quality of life in older patients with ovarian epithelial, primary peritoneal cavity, or fallopian tube cancer [32]. Patients and their physicians decided between regimen I (carboplatin AUC 5 and paclitaxel 135 mg/m^2 plus GCSF, every 3 weeks) and regimen II (carboplatin AUC 5 every 3 weeks) for 4 cycles either after primary surgery or as neoadjuvant chemotherapy. Two hundred and eight evaluable patients were enrolled onto regimen I ($n = 149$) or regimen II ($n = 59$). Completion rates were high (92 % versus 75 %). In the multivariate analysis, the inability to complete four cycles of chemotherapy was associated with regimen II ($p < 0.001$), neoadjuvant chemotherapy ($p = 0.024$), and

Table 5.2 Final results of age-specific prospective trials in elderly women with ovarian cancer treated with first-line chemotherapy

	First author	Inclusion period	Chemotherapy regimen	N	Age (median, range in years)	PS ≥2 (%)	TCR (%)	OS (months)
FAG 1	Freyer G.	1997–2000	Carboplatin AUC5-cyclophosphamide Every 3 weeks	83	76 [70–90]	44	72	21.6
FAG 2	Tredan O.	1997–2000	Carboplatin-paclitaxel Every 3 weeks	72	75 [70–89]	26	68.5	25.9
FAG 3	Falandry C.	2007–2010	Carboplatin AUC 5 Every 3 weeks	111	79 [71–93]	47	73.9	17.4
MITO 5	Pignata S.	2003–2005	Weekly carboplatin AUC2-paclitaxel 60 mg/m^2	26	77 [70–84]	0	65	32

FAG "Femme AGée" (elderly woman in English), N number of enrolled patients, PS performance status, TCR treatment completion rate, OS overall survival limited social activities ($p=0.034$), but not IADLs ($p=0.2$). In both regimens, patient reported outcomes improved over time with cumulative chemotherapy cycles and at a similar pace. A third arm, evaluating weekly paclitaxel 60 mg/m^2 and carboplatin AUC 5 every 3 weeks, was added to the study. Final results are awaited (ClinicalTrials.gov identifier NCT01366183).

Other strategies have been evaluated in retrospective analysis such as reduced doses or addition of a third cytotoxic agent.

Reduced doses were evaluated in a retrospective cohort [33]. Patients received carboplatin AUC 4–5 and paclitaxel 135 mg/m^2. Twenty-six patients treated with reduced doses (RD) were compared to 74 patients treated with standard doses (SD). Median age was 77.0 in the RD group. Incidence of grade 3–4 neutropenia was higher in the SD group (54.1 % versus 19.2 %; $p=0.002$). SD patients were more likely to experience cumulative toxicity ($p=0.003$) and required delays in treatment schedule ($p=0.05$). There were no differences in PFS or OS between cohorts.

Compared with standard paclitaxel and carboplatin, **addition of a third cytotoxic agent** such as gemcitabine, topotecan, or pegylated liposomal doxorubicin (PLD) provided a small benefit in PFS (1 month) but a shorter OS (37 versus 45 months) and increased toxicity (cytopenias and neurotoxicity) in a retrospective analysis of 620 elderly patients included in the Gynecologic Oncology Group (GOG) 182 phase III trial [24, 34].

Intraperitoneal Chemotherapy

Even though advantage in survival has been demonstrated with intraperitoneal chemotherapy compared to intravenous chemotherapy in three randomized trials [35–37], it has not been fully adopted, particularly in Europe, due to concerns about the higher rate of toxicities and technical difficulties.

Furthermore, its role in the elderly is still not quite clear. A small proportion of elderly patients were included in the three trials mentioned above. In the GOG 172 trial [36], 13 % of the patients were older than 70 years, but older patients had a good functional status in 92 % of cases, and less than half of them were able to complete ≥4 cycles due to toxicities.

Although one report suggested the elderly could tolerate intraperitoneal chemotherapy [38], another small report suggested critical outcomes following interval cytoreduction and hyperthermic intraperitoneal chemotherapy (HIPEC) with 78 % grade I–IV toxicities.

Addition of an Antiangiogenic Agent Such as Bevacizumab

Concerning the addition of antiangiogenic agents to front-line chemotherapy, no age-specific trials are available. Yet, in the GOG 218 randomized phase III trial, the effect in terms of improvement of PFS was seen consistently in all the prognostic subgroups including the age subgroup [39]. However, bevacizumab use requires more caution in the elderly due to more frequent grade ≥ 3 toxicity and more vascular events (8.5 % arterial thromboembolic events in patients older than 65 compared to 2.9 % in younger patients) [40]. Comorbidities and associated risk factors such as personal history of hypertension, stroke or transient ischemic attack, etc. must be carefully evaluated prior to prescription, and patients must be closely monitored.

Neoadjuvant Chemotherapy

Use of neoadjuvant therapy has increased over time particularly in old and frail patients [41]. Indeed, cytoreductive surgery (CRS) is associated with substantial postoperative morbidity [42], and there are several issues concerning chemotherapy delivery following surgery with significant delays in the initiation of chemotherapy [43]. Neoadjuvant chemotherapy, on the other hand, reduces the burden of surgical procedure, increases rates of optimal CRS [44], and reduces perioperative morbidity and mortality [45].

To address this issue, the European Organization for Research and Treatment of Cancer has developed a randomized trial (EORTC 55971) comparing neoadjuvant chemotherapy followed by interval debulking surgery with primary debulking surgery followed by chemotherapy [46]. This non-inferiority trial showed similar overall survival, which was the primary endpoint, with a median OS of 29 months in the primary surgery group and 30 months in the neoadjuvant-chemotherapy group. The hazard ratio for death (intention-to-treat analysis) in the neoadjuvant-chemotherapy group as compared with the primary surgery group was 0.98 (90%IC [0.84–1.13], $p = 0.01$ for non-inferiority). Besides, postoperative deaths were reported in 2.5 % versus 0.7 % and infections in 8.1 % versus 1.7 % in the primary surgery group versus the neoadjuvant-chemotherapy group, respectively. Exploratory analyses did not show differences in benefit by age [47]. Similarly, in an analysis of 9587 women ≥ 65 years of age (SEER-Medicare database), survival with neoadjuvant chemotherapy did not differ significantly from primary surgery (HR = 1.04; 95 % CI = 0.67–1.60) [41].

However, in the EORTC 55971 trial [47], patients with stage IIIC and less extensive metastatic tumors showed greater survival with primary surgery, while patients with stage IV disease and large metastatic tumors had higher survival with neoadjuvant chemotherapy.

Following the results of this trial [46] and its exploratory analysis [47], a lot of controversy on the role of neoadjuvant chemotherapy and primary debulking in advanced ovarian cancer emerged. Specialists suggest that neoadjuvant chemotherapy followed by interval debulking surgery should be limited to selected patients such as patients with high initial tumor burden FIGO stage III OC or FIGO stage IV OC or frail patients ≥ 75 [48–50] and that primary surgery, with a complete resection objective, should remain the standard in other cases. Indeed, patients who gain most benefit from surgery are those with no residual disease at the end of the procedure. Therefore, to determine the best therapeutic strategy between primary surgery and neoadjuvant chemotherapy followed by interval CRS, the likelihood that surgery results in R0 resection should be evaluated. In this regard, French specialists agree that primary laparoscopic evaluation should be performed in order to predict R0 resection and to avoid unnecessary surgical procedures [51]. In a recent systematic review [52], even though laparoscopic evaluating showed promising results in predicting resectability, no firm conclusions could be drawn as too few and heterogeneous studies were included in the analysis. In this regard, a multicenter randomized controlled trial, LapOvCa-trial [53], is actually ongoing to identify the role of laparoscopy in predicting the result of primary CRS in advanced ovarian cancer patients (Netherlands Trial Register number NTR2644).

Conclusion

Identification of vulnerable elderly patients is crucial to overcome interindividual variability in first-line chemotherapy tolerance and therefore efficacy. While standard first-line chemotherapy with 3-weekly carboplatin AUC 5 mg/mL/min and paclitaxel 175 mg/m^2 in advanced ovarian cancer may be feasible in selected elderly patients such as those included in prospective trials, in a wider selection of patients $\geq$70, as this is the case in everyday practice, the standard carboplatin-paclitaxel regimen has shown an excess of toxicity and led to premature treatment stopping. For elderly patients thought to be vulnerable and at high risk of toxicity with the standard 3-weekly carboplatin-paclitaxel regimen, other options are commonly used: carboplatin as a single agent and carboplatin-paclitaxel regimen in a weekly schedule for both drugs. To date, there is no randomized trial to give practitioners some evidence on how to select patients who could benefit from one or the other regimen described above. The GINECO has therefore designed EWOC-1 (Elderly Women Ovarian Cancer), an international multicenter randomized phase II trial, to compare three different regimens: paclitaxel + carboplatin every 3 weeks, single-agent carboplatin every 3 weeks, and weekly paclitaxel and carboplatin in a selected population of vulnerable elderly patients (defined using the geriatric vulnerability score described above) (ClinicalTrials.gov identifier NCT02001272). The primary outcome of this trial is the treatment success defined as the ability to deliver six courses of chemotherapy without premature termination for progression, death, or unacceptable toxicity. Secondary outcome measures include feasibility, OS, PFS, quality of life, safety, tolerability, and aging biomarkers. This trial is actually recruiting and primary outcome measure will be carried out around May 2018.

In the future, a better understanding of the place of neoadjuvant chemotherapy and bevacizumab and the sequence of treatment will be needed as these issues remain unresolved in older ovarian cancer patients.

References

1. Ferlay J, Soerjomataram I, Dikshit R, Eser S, Mathers C, Rebelo M, et al. Cancer incidence and mortality worldwide: sources, methods and major patterns in GLOBOCAN 2012. Int J Cancer J Int du Cancer. 2015;136(5):E359–86.
2. Oberaigner W, Minicozzi P, Bielska-Lasota M, Allemani C, de Angelis R, Mangone L, et al. Survival for ovarian cancer in Europe: the across-country variation did not shrink in the past decade. Acta Oncol. 2012;51(4):441–53.
3. Yancik R, Ries LA. Cancer in older persons: an international issue in an aging world. Semin Oncol. 2004;31(2):128–36.
4. Lowe KA, Chia VM, Taylor A, O'Malley C, Kelsh M, Mohamed M, et al. An international assessment of ovarian cancer incidence and mortality. Gynecol Oncol. 2013;130(1):107–14.
5. Yancik R. Ovarian cancer. Age contrasts in incidence, histology, disease stage at diagnosis, and mortality. Cancer. 1993;71(2 Suppl):517–23.
6. Berchuck A, Kohler MF, Boente MP, Rodriguez GC, Whitaker RS, Bast RC, Bast Jr RC. GROWTH regulation and transformation of ovarian epithelium. Cancer. 1993;71(2 Suppl):545–51.
7. Zola P, Ferrero A. Is carboplatin-paclitaxel combination the standard treatment of elderly ovarian cancer patients? Ann Oncol. 2007;18(2):213–4.
8. Bruchim I, Altaras M, Fishman A. Age contrasts in clinical characteristics and pattern of care in patients with epithelial ovarian cancer. Gynecol Oncol. 2002;86(3):274–8.
9. Hurria A, Cirrincione CT, Muss HB, Kornblith AB, Barry W, Artz AS, et al. Implementing a geriatric assessment in cooperative group clinical cancer trials: CALGB 360401. J Clin Oncol. 2011;29(10):1290–6.
10. Hurria A, Togawa K, Mohile SG, Owusu C, Klepin HD, Gross CP, et al. Predicting chemotherapy toxicity in older adults with cancer: a prospective multicenter study. J Clin Oncol. 2011;29(25):3457–65.
11. Freyer G, Geay JF, Touzet S, Provencal J, Weber B, Jacquin JP, et al. Comprehensive geriatric assessment predicts tolerance to chemotherapy and survival in elderly patients with advanced ovarian carcinoma: a GINECO study. Ann Oncol. 2005;16(11):1795–800.
12. Falandry C, Weber B, Savoye AM, Tinquaut F, Tredan O, Sevin E, et al. Development of a geriatric vulnerability score in elderly patients with advanced ovarian cancer treated with first-line carboplatin: a GINECO prospective trial. Ann Oncol. 2013;24(11):2808–13.
13. Piccart MJ, Bertelsen K, James K, Cassidy J, Mangioni C, Simonsen E, et al. Randomized intergroup trial of cisplatin-paclitaxel versus cisplatin-cyclophosphamide in women with advanced epithelial ovarian cancer: three-year results. J Natl Cancer Inst. 2000;92(9):699–708.
14. du Bois A, Luck HJ, Meier W, Adams HP, Mobus V, Costa S, et al. A randomized clinical trial of cisplatin/paclitaxel versus carboplatin/paclitaxel as first-line treatment of ovarian cancer. J Natl Cancer Inst. 2003;95(17):1320–9.
15. Ozols RF, Bundy BN, Greer BE, Fowler JM, Clarke-Pearson D, Burger RA, et al. Phase III trial of carboplatin and paclitaxel compared with cisplatin and paclitaxel in patients with optimally resected stage III ovarian cancer: a Gynecologic Oncology Group study. J Clin Oncol. 2003;21(17):3194–200.
16. Mcguire WP, Hoskins WJ, Brady MF, Kucera PR, Partridge EE, Look KY, et al. Cyclophosphamide and cisplatin versus paclitaxel and cisplatin: a phase III randomized trial in patients with suboptimal stage III/IV ovarian cancer (from the Gynecologic Oncology Group). Semin Oncol. 1996;23(5 Suppl 12):40–7.
17. Swenerton K, Jeffrey J, Stuart G, Roy M, Krepart G, Carmichael J, et al. Cisplatin-cyclophosphamide versus carboplatin-cyclophosphamide in advanced ovarian cancer: a randomized phase III study of the National Cancer Institute of Canada Clinical Trials Group. J Clin Oncol. 1992;10(5):718–26.

18. Hershman D, Jacobson JS, Mcbride R, Mitra N, Sundararajan V, Grann VR, et al. Effectiveness of platinum-based chemotherapy among elderly patients with advanced ovarian cancer. Gynecol Oncol. 2004;94(2):540–9.
19. Sundararajan V, Hershman D, Grann VR, Jacobson JS, Neugut AI. Variations in the use of chemotherapy for elderly patients with advanced ovarian cancer: a population-based study. J Clin Oncol. 2002;20(1):173–8.
20. Fairfield KM, Murray K, Lucas FL, Wierman HR, Earle CC, Trimble EL, et al. Completion of adjuvant chemotherapy and use of health services for older women with epithelial ovarian cancer. J Clin Oncol. 2011;29(29):3921–6.
21. Maas HA, Kruitwagen RF, Lemmens VE, Goey SH, Janssen-Heijnen ML. The influence of age and co-morbidity on treatment and prognosis of ovarian cancer: a population-based study. Gynecol Oncol. 2005;97(1):104–9.
22. Gajra A, Klepin HD, Feng T, Tew WP, Mohile SG, Owusu C, et al. Predictors of chemotherapy dose reduction at first cycle in patients age 65years and older with solid tumors. J Geriatr Oncol. 2015;6(2):133–40.
23. Ceccaroni M, D'agostino G, Ferrandina G, Gadducci A, di Vagno G, Pignata S, et al. Gynecological malignancies in elderly patients: is age 70 a limit to standard-dose chemotherapy? An Italian retrospective toxicity multicentric study. Gynecol Oncol. 2002;85(3):445–50.
24. Tew WP, Java J, Chi D, Menzin A, Lovecchio JL, Bookman MA, et al. Treatment outcomes for older women with advanced ovarian cancer: results from a phase III clinical trial (GOG182). J Clin Oncol. 2010;28:15s. suppl; abstr 5030.
25. Hilpert F, du BOIS A, Greimel ER, Hedderich J, Krause G, Venhoff L, et al. Feasibility, toxicity and quality of life of first-line chemotherapy with platinum/paclitaxel in elderly patients aged > or =70 years with advanced ovarian cancer – a study by the AGO-OVAR Germany. Ann Oncol. 2007;18(2):282–7.
26. Balducci L, Extermann M. Management of cancer in the older person: a practical approach. Oncologist. 2000;5(3):224–37.
27. Tredan O, Geay JF, Touzet S, Delva R, Weber B, Cretin J, et al. Carboplatin/cyclophosphamide or carboplatin/paclitaxel in elderly patients with advanced ovarian cancer? Analysis of two consecutive trials from the Groupe d'Investigateurs Nationaux pour l'Etude des Cancers Ovariens. Ann Oncol. 2007;18(2):256–62.
28. Pignata S, Monfardini S. Single agents should be administered in preference to combination chemotherapy for the treatment of patients over 70 years of age with advanced ovarian carcinoma. Eur J Cancer. 2000;36(7):817–20.
29. International Collaborative Ovarian Neoplasm Group. Paclitaxel plus carboplatin versus standard chemotherapy with either single-agent carboplatin or cyclophosphamide, doxorubicin, and cisplatin in women with ovarian cancer: the ICON3 randomised trial. Lancet. 2002;360(9332):505–15.
30. Pignata S, Breda E, Scambia G, Pisano C, Zagonel V, Lorusso D, et al. A phase II study of weekly carboplatin and paclitaxel as first-line treatment of elderly patients with advanced ovarian cancer. A Multicentre Italian Trial in Ovarian cancer (MITO-5) study. Crit Rev Oncol Hematol. 2008;66(3):229–36.
31. Pignata S, Scambia G, Katsaros D, Gallo C, Pujade-Lauraine E, de Placido S, et al. Carboplatin plus paclitaxel once a week versus every 3 weeks in patients with advanced ovarian cancer (MITO-7): a randomised, multicentre, open-label, phase 3 trial. Lancet Oncol. 2014;15(4):396–405.
32. von Gruenigen VE, Huang H, Tew W, Hurria AH, Lankes H, Disilvestro PA, et al. 3Geriatric assessment and tolerance to chemotherapy in elderly women with ovarian, primary peritoneal or fallopian tube cancer: a Gynecologic Oncology Group study. Gynecol Oncol. 2014;134(2):438–40.
33. Fader AN, von Gruenigen V, Gibbons H, Abushahin F, Starks D, Markman M, et al. Improved tolerance of primary chemotherapy with reduced-dose carboplatin and paclitaxel in elderly ovarian cancer patients. Gynecol Oncol. 2008;109(1):33–8.

34. Bookman MA, Brady MF, Mcguire WP, Harper PG, Alberts DS, Friedlander M, et al. Evaluation of new platinum-based treatment regimens in advanced-stage ovarian cancer: a Phase III Trial of the Gynecologic Cancer Intergroup. J Clin Oncol. 2009;27(9):1419–25.
35. Alberts DS, Liu PY, Hannigan EV, O'toole R, Williams SD, Young JA, et al. Intraperitoneal cisplatin plus intravenous cyclophosphamide versus intravenous cisplatin plus intravenous cyclophosphamide for stage III ovarian cancer. N Engl J Med. 1996;335(26):1950–5.
36. Armstrong DK, Bundy B, Wenzel L, Huang HQ, Baergen R, Lele S, et al. Intraperitoneal cisplatin and paclitaxel in ovarian cancer. N Engl J Med. 2006;354(1):34–43.
37. Markman M, Bundy BN, Alberts DS, Fowler JM, Clark-Pearson DL, Carson LF, et al. Phase III trial of standard-dose intravenous cisplatin plus paclitaxel versus moderately high-dose carboplatin followed by intravenous paclitaxel and Intraperitoneal cisplatin in small-volume stage III ovarian carcinoma: an intergroup study of the Gynecologic Oncology Group, Southwestern Oncology Group, and Eastern Cooperative Oncology Group. J Clin Oncol. 2001;19(4):1001–7.
38. Tew WP, O'Cearbhaill R, Zhou Q, Thaler H, Konner J, Hensley ML, et al. Intraperitoneal chemotherapy in older women with epithelial ovarian cancer. J Clin Oncol. 2009;27:[abstr ♯5541].
39. Burger RA, Brady MF, Bookman MA, Fleming GF, Monk BJ, Huang H, et al. Incorporation of Bevacizumab in the primary treatment of ovarian cancer. N Engl J Med. 2011;365(26):2473–83.
40. Mohile SG, Hardt M, Tew W, Owusu C, Klepin H, Gross C, et al. Toxicity of Bevacizumab in combination with chemotherapy in older patients. Oncologist. 2013;18(4):408–14.
41. Wright JD, Ananth CV, Tsui J, Glied SA, Burke WM, Lu YS. Comparative effectiveness of upfront treatment strategies in elderly women with ovarian cancer. Cancer. 2014;120(8):1246–54.
42. Fotopoulou C, Savvatis K, Steinhagen-Thiessen E, Bahra M, Lichtenegger W, Sehouli J. Primary radical surgery in elderly patients with epithelial ovarian cancer: analysis of surgical outcome and long-term survival. Int J Gynecol Cancer. 2010;20(1):34–40.
43. Wright JD, Herzog TJ, Neugut AI, Burke WM, Lu YS, Lewin SN. Effect of radical cytoreductive surgery on omission and delay of chemotherapy for advanced-stage ovarian cancer. Obstet Gynecol. 2012;120(4):871–81.
44. Kang S, Nam BH. Does neoadjuvant chemotherapy increase optimal cytoreduction rate in advanced ovarian cancer? Meta-analysis of 21 studies. Ann Surg Oncol. 2009;16(8):2315–20.
45. Mclean KA, Shah CA, Thompson SA, Gray HJ, Swensen RE, Goff BA. Ovarian cancer in the elderly: outcomes with neoadjuvant chemotherapy or primary cytoreduction. Gynecol Oncol. 2010;118(1):43–6.
46. Vergote I, Trope CG, Amant F, Kristensen GB, Ehlen T, Johnson N, et al. Neoadjuvant chemotherapy or primary surgery in stage IIIC or IV ovarian cancer. N Engl J Med. 2010;363(10):943–53.
47. van Meurs HS, Tajik P, Hof MH, Vergote I, Kenter GG, Mol BW, et al. Which patients benefit most from primary surgery or neoadjuvant chemotherapy in stage IIIC or IV ovarian cancer? An exploratory analysis of the European Organisation for Research and Treatment of Cancer 55971 randomised trial. Eur J Cancer. 2013;49(15):3191–201.
48. Aletti GD, Eisenhauer EL, Santillan A, Axtell A, Aletti G, Holschneider C, et al. Identification of patient groups at highest risk from traditional approach to ovarian cancer treatment. Gynecol Oncol. 2011;120(1):23–8.
49. Thrall MM, Goff BA, Symons RG, Flum DR, Gray HJ. Thirty-day mortality after primary cytoreductive surgery for advanced ovarian cancer in the elderly. Obstet Gynecol. 2011;118(3):537–47.
50. Vergote I, du Bois A, Amant F, Heitz F, Leunen K, Harter P. Neoadjuvant chemotherapy in advanced ovarian cancer: on what do we agree and disagree? Gynecol Oncol. 2013;128(1):6–11.

51. Falandry C, Fabbro M, Lesoin A, Guerin O, Kurtz JE. 1ères recommandations sur le cancer de l'ovaire. Nice-St Paul de Vence 2012. Cancer de l'ovaire de la patiente âgée. Onko+. 2013;5(2):40.
52. Rutten MJ, Leeflang MM, Kenter GG, Mol BW, Buist M. Laparoscopy for diagnosing resectability of disease in patients with advanced ovarian cancer. Cochrane Database Syst Rev. 2014;2, CD009786.
53. Rutten MJ, Gaarenstroom KN, van Gorp T, van Meurs HS, Arts HJ, Bossuyt PM, et al. Laparoscopy to predict the result of primary cytoreductive surgery in advanced ovarian cancer patients (LapOvCa-trial): a multicentre randomized controlled study. BMC Cancer. 2012;12:31.

Chemotherapy for Recurrent Ovarian Cancer in the Elderly Patients

6

Jean-Emmanuel Kurtz and Laure de Cock

Contents

Introduction

It is now widely acknowledged that the elderly represent a significant proportion of advanced ovarian cancer patients and that age is negatively linked to the use of chemotherapy [1] [2]. Despite having been neglected and excluded from clinical trials in the past, these patients may at present benefit from the same advances in cancer care as their younger counterparts do provided geriatric assessment including comorbidities is taken into account [3, 4]. Indeed, age itself is not a poor prognostic factor, at least for frontline chemotherapy [5]. Owing to the advances that have been achieved in the care of elderly patients either for surgery or medical therapy, the lower boundary for old age has evolved from 65 years old (that is

J.-E. Kurtz, MD, PHD (✉) • L. de Cock, MD
Service d'Oncologie et d'Hématologie, Hôpitaux Universitaires de Strasbourg, 1 Av Molière, 67098 Strasbourg, France
e-mail: j-emmanuel.kurtz@chru-strasbourg.fr

© Springer International Publishing Switzerland 2016
G. Freyer (ed.), *Ovarian Cancer in Elderly Patients*,
DOI 10.1007/978-3-319-23588-2_6

currently considered as absolutely inappropriate) to 70 and 75 years old. Indeed, an international effort has been undertaken to better handle elderly cancer patients, with the development of oncogeriatrics and the incorporation of geriatric issues in oncology trials. In France, the different iterations of the French *plan cancer*, besides the nationwide implementation of coordination units in oncogeriatrics supported by the National Institute for Cancer (INCa) as well as the efforts of collaborative groups such as GINECO, have put to the foreground the problematic of ovarian cancer in the elderly. Of note, although most of the effort was put on the care of newly diagnosed patients with trials focusing on frontline chemotherapy, there is a need for exploring the benefits and pitfalls of salvage therapy in relapsing patients as at least second and third lines of chemotherapy may increase survival [6]. This is indeed a relevant issue, as most of patients with advanced disease at diagnosis will experience a relapse, and as ovarian cancer incidence peaks in the 70s, we need to define strategies of care that fits well to the elderly relapsing patients.

All Recurrent Patients Are Not the Same: Refractory and Resistant Versus Platinum-Sensitive Disease

The medical history of recurrent ovarian cancer is dominated by the relapse status toward prior platinum salts exposure. Either in young or old age, there is no getting away from the facts, and patients with late relapse (>6 months after last platinum dose), characterized as *platinum sensitive*, have a reasonable chance to respond again to the same drugs and are of best prognosis. Conversely, patient with early relapse (<6 months) or those progressing during therapy or within the next 4 weeks fall into the *platinum-resistant* and *platinum- refractory* groups, respectively [7–10]. As in the young patients, the latter category has such as dismal prognosis that we have limited options if any that may apply to the elderly patients. Conversely, there is room for exploring the care of both platinum-sensitive and platinum-resistant patients with an integrated approach that fits well the elderly, mixing efficacy, and tolerance/quality of life issues.

Current Option for Medical Care of Ovarian Cancer Relapse: Do They Apply to the Elderly Patients?

As it was shown that elderly people benefited as much as the young for optimal frontline therapy (when feasible, as established if necessary through an oncogeriatric assessment), it is tempting to apply standard relapse protocols to the elderly. However, one must acknowledge that elderly patients may, at the time of relapse, not have fully recovered from frontline therapy side effects, notably neuropathy. Moreover, they are also prone to having a decreased functional reserve because of initial surgery and chemotherapy, besides being sometimes less willing to reiterate multiple cycles of chemotherapy.

Platinum-Sensitive Patients

The current guidelines for the care of advanced ovarian cancer recommend that patients with platinum-sensitive recurrence be re-challenged with platinum salts [8, 10]. There is still some debate to whether platinum single-agent or a platinum-based doublet should be given to elderly ovarian cancer patients in relapse. In the SOCRATES study, Pignata et al. retrospectively reported the outcomes of elderly patients treated with platinum salts in late recurrence. Among the 94 elderly patients, more received single-agent carboplatin as compared to the young, presumably due to the fear of side effects such as neurotoxicity and myelotoxicity. Moreover, elderly patients in the SOCRATES study experienced more treatment delays and dose reductions than the young and unexpectedly a poorer response to therapy [11]. Regardless of age, the combination of paclitaxel (T) and carboplatin (C) is a standard of care in platinum-sensitive relapse. To explore a possibly less toxic schedule, TC was compared to the carboplatin and pegylated liposomal doxorubicin (PLD) combination in the CALYPSO study [12]. Interestingly, the CALYPSO study enrolled patients of all ages, and a sub-analysis was performed to analyze the elderly population ($\geq$70 years old). This leads to the findings that (i) the C-PLD was safe and had a better tolerability profile than C-T in the elderly, particularly regarding neuropathy (that negatively impacted quality of life in the C-T arm) and alopecia, and (ii) older patients were exposed to a higher risk of neuropathy, thus experiencing less allergic reactions (Table 6.1) [13]. Indeed, these differences make sense in the setting of elderly patients, where combined sensory neuropathy, arthralgias/myalgias, and hand-foot syndrome are likely to jeopardize patients' activity and autonomy. Although the sub-study was not designed to detect survival differences, PFS was similar in both arms with 11.6 and 10.3 months in the C-PLD and C-T

Table 6.1 Summary of C-PLD vs. C-T tolerance in elderly patients (Adapted from [13])

	C-PLD	C-P	p
Febrile neutropenia			
None	100	94	0.038
Present	0	6	
Alopecia			
None	89	14	<0.001
Partial/complete	11	86	
Sensory neuropathy			
Grade 0–1	90	64	<0.001
Grade 2–3	10	36	
Hand-foot syndrome			
Grade 0–1	86	98	<0.001
Grade 2–3	14	2	
Arthralgia/myalgia			
Grade 0–1	97	78	<0.001
Grade 2–3	3	22	

arms, respectively. Moreover, with the same limitations, C-PLD performed similarly in young and elderly patients. Of note, elderly patients enrolled in this study were probably selected, but oncologists have incorporated the C-PLD schedule in routine practice.

The incorporation of bevacizumab in treatment schedules for recurrent, platinum-sensitive disease has been assessed in the OCEANS trial that enrolled patients, regardless of age [14]. In this trial, bevacizumab was compared to placebo, combined to gemcitabine and carboplatin. Indeed, 35 % and 38 % of these were older than 65 in the bevacizumab and placebo arm, respectively, although more accurate data toward age distribution is not available. The trial concluded to the superiority of the bevacizumab-containing arm, with a side-effect spectrum marked by hypertension and chemotherapy-induced myelotoxicity. Efficacy analysis in the >65 years old population showed again a favorable PFS hazard ratio toward bevacizumab (HR = 0.50, CI95% 0.34–0.72). Although shown feasible in selected patients to be enrolled into a phase III trial, it is unclear whether the carboplatin-gemcitabine chemotherapy backbone suits all elderly patients, due to its toxicity profile. The ongoing AGO 2.21 study (NCT01837251), currently recruiting adult patients regardless of age, compares the CALYPSO and OCEANS schedules, both in combination with bevacizumab. The study has a PFS primary end point, and secondary end point includes safety and quality of life. Hopefully, some analysis will be undertaken to explore these issues in the elderly patient subpopulation.

Platinum-Refractory and Resistant Patients

As discussed above, platinum-resistant and refractory patients have a poor prognosis and, at the time of recurrence, have usually not recovered from initial weight loss and side effects of frontline therapy. Hence they often present with fatigue, impaired functional capacity, and for the elderly, a high risk of lack of autonomy. It is not surprising that in this setting, performance status (despite its limitations) is a key prognosis factor when considering salvage chemotherapy. Yet, given the very poor prognosis of platinum-refractory patient, most of the published data focus onto platinum-resistant ovarian cancer. In a retrospective series of 102 patients, Gronlund et al. found that three prognostic factors independently impact overall survival: performance status at initial and salvage therapy and response to second-line therapy [15]. Since no combination chemotherapy has proven superiority over single-agent therapy in this setting, therapeutic options include gemcitabine, pegylated liposomal doxorubicin, topotecan, and weekly paclitaxel [10]. Despite there is no trial specifically assessing these drugs in elderly recurrent ovarian cancer, some phase III trials included elderly patients and concluded to similar efficacy with acceptable, albeit different, toxicity profiles [16, 17]. More recently, the AURELIA trial assessed the combination of bevacizumab with any of these drugs versus single-agent chemotherapy [18]. Again, the trial included elderly patients, and concluded to the superiority of the bevacizumab arm. A post-hoc analysis of the AURELIA study has been undertaken, to explore the outcomes of elderly versus young patients in the study, although the cutoff boundary for old age was only 65 [19]. Nevertheless, 133 patients aged ≥65 years old were compared to 227 young (<65) patients. The benefit from adding bevacizumab was also found in the elderly subgroup, with a PFS hazard ratio of 0.47 (CI95% 0.32-0.70). Moreover, no major difference in safety was observed, despite that hypertension was more frequent in elderly patients and in those receiving bevacizumab, suggesting a favorable risk/benefit ratio in this population.

Conclusion

During the last decade, there has been an unprecedented effort to a better care of elderly ovarian cancer patient. However, most of the published data or ongoing studies have focused on frontline therapy, including the treatment tailoring to elderly patients' vulnerabilities. Since it appears that age does not preclude the efficacy of first-line therapy and second- and third-line treatments are associated with a survival benefit, elderly patients should not be excluded from recurrent disease trials. As well, they should benefit from a careful pretreatment assessment to detect limitations that may render the treatment harmful, especially in the setting of platinum-resistant disease. Finally, it is mandatory that future trials in this setting not only focus onto efficacy data, but also assess patients' reported outcomes as well as quality of life.

References

1. Thigpen T, Brady MF, Omura GA, et al. Age as a prognostic factor in ovarian carcinoma. The Gynecologic Oncology Group experience. Cancer. 1993;71:606–14.
2. Uyar D, Frasure HE, Markman M, von Gruenigen VE. Treatment patterns by decade of life in elderly women (> or =70 years of age) with ovarian cancer. Gynecol Oncol. 2005; 98:403–8.
3. Freyer G, Tew WP, Moore KN. Treatment and trials: ovarian cancer in older women. Am Soc Clin Oncol Educ Book. 2013:227–35. doi: 10.1200/EdBook_AM.2013.33.227.
4. Chia VM, O'Malley CD, Danese MD, et al. Prevalence and incidence of comorbidities in elderly women with ovarian cancer. Gynecol Oncol. 2013;129:346–52.
5. Eisenhauer EL, Tew WP, Levine DA, et al. Response and outcomes in elderly patients with stages IIIC-IV ovarian cancer receiving platinum-taxane chemotherapy. Gynecol Oncol. 2007;106:381–7.
6. Hanker LC, Loibl S, Burchardi N, et al. The impact of second to sixth line therapy on survival of relapsed ovarian cancer after primary taxane/platinum-based therapy. Ann Oncol. 2012;23:2605–12.
7. Mcguire WP, Ozols RF. Chemotherapy of advanced ovarian cancer. Semin Oncol. 1998;25:340–8.
8. Thigpen JT, Vance RB, Khansur T. Second-line chemotherapy for recurrent carcinoma of the ovary. Cancer. 1993;71:1559–64.
9. Friedlander M, Trimble E, Tinker A, et al. Clinical trials in recurrent ovarian cancer. Int J Gynecol Cancer. 2011;21:771–5.
10. Ledermann JA, Raja FA, Fotopoulou C, et al. Newly diagnosed and relapsed epithelial ovarian carcinoma: ESMO Clinical Practice Guidelines for diagnosis, treatment and follow-up. Ann Oncol. 2013;24 Suppl 6:vi24–32.

11. Pignata S, Ferrandina G, Scarfone G, et al. Poor outcome of elderly patients with platinum-sensitive recurrent ovarian cancer: results from the SOCRATES retrospective study. Crit Rev Oncol Hematol. 2009;71:233–41.
12. Pujade-Lauraine E, Wagner U, Aavall-Lundqvist E, et al. Pegylated liposomal Doxorubicin and Carboplatin compared with Paclitaxel and Carboplatin for patients with platinum-sensitive ovarian cancer in late relapse. J Clin Oncol. 2010;28:3323–9.
13. Kurtz JE, Kaminsky MC, Floquet A, et al. Ovarian cancer in elderly patients: carboplatin and pegylated liposomal doxorubicin versus carboplatin and paclitaxel in late relapse: a Gynecologic Cancer Intergroup (GCIG) CALYPSO sub-study. Ann Oncol. 2011;22:2417–23.
14. Aghajanian C, Blank SV, Goff BA, et al. OCEANS: a randomized, double-blind, placebo-controlled phase III trial of chemotherapy with or without bevacizumab in patients with platinum-sensitive recurrent epithelial ovarian, primary peritoneal, or fallopian tube cancer. J Clin Oncol. 2012;30:2039–45.
15. Gronlund B, Hogdall C, Hansen HH, Engelholm SA. Performance status rather than age is the key prognostic factor in second-line treatment of elderly patients with epithelial ovarian carcinoma. Cancer. 2002;94:1961–7.
16. Mutch DG, Orlando M, Goss T, et al. Randomized phase III trial of gemcitabine compared with pegylated liposomal doxorubicin in patients with platinum-resistant ovarian cancer. J Clin Oncol. 2007;25:2811–8.
17. Gordon AN, Fleagle JT, Guthrie D, et al. Recurrent epithelial ovarian carcinoma: a randomized phase III study of pegylated liposomal doxorubicin versus topotecan. J Clin Oncol. 2001;19:3312–22.
18. Pujade-Lauraine E, Hilpert F, Weber B, et al. Bevacizumab combined with chemotherapy for platinum-resistant recurrent ovarian cancer: the AURELIA open-label randomized phase III trial. J Clin Oncol. 2014;32(13):1302–8.
19. Sorio R, Roemer-Becuwe C, Hilpert F, et al. Effect of bevacizumab and chemotherapy in elderly patients: subgroup analysis of the AURELIA open-label randomised phase III trial in platinum-resistant recurrent ovarian cancer. Int J Gynecol Cancer. 2013;23:136.

Management of Antiangiogenic Agents

7

Olivier Trédan and Isabelle Ray-Coquard

Contents

Introduction

Vascular endothelial growth factor (VEGF) plays a major role in ovarian cancers, especially in stimulating endothelial cell proliferation, migration, and survival, as well as in modifying expression of adhesion molecules and vascular permeability. Thus, one of the etiologies of malignant peritoneal effusions (i.e., in ovarian cancer) may be attributed to an increased permeability of serous membrane lining vessels. VEGF increases capillary leakage by opening the endothelial intracellular junctions and by inducing fenestration development in the endothelia. Because of the role of VEGF in the physiological and in the pathophysiological angiogenesis, targeting

O. Trédan (✉) • I. Ray-Coquard
Centre Léon Bérard et Groupe GINECO, Lyon, France
e-mail: olivier.tredan@lyon.unicancer.fr

© Springer International Publishing Switzerland 2016
G. Freyer (ed.), *Ovarian Cancer in Elderly Patients*,
DOI 10.1007/978-3-319-23588-2_7

VEGF may cause serious adverse vascular events, such as venous/arterial thrombo-embolic events or bleeding. Furthermore, VEGF inhibition results in hyaline depos-its in renal capillaries, glomerulopathy, as well as endothelial production of nitric oxide, leading to hypertension and proteinuria [1].

Specific characteristics of elderly patients (who may have cardiovascular comor-bidities and/or co-medications) may increase the risk of anti-VEGF treatment side effects. However, elderly patients are underrepresented in clinical trials assessing anti-VEGF treatment safety and efficacy. This may be due to the concerns of increased toxic effects in case of advanced age and/or comorbidities.

Since VEGF is expressed in the majority of ovarian cancers, bevacizumab, a humanized monoclonal antibody that targets VEGF, has been tested in various lines of treatment in ovarian cancer patients. This is the first antiangiogenic agent approved by the European Medicines Agency (EMEA) in combination with che-motherapy (carboplatin/paclitaxel) as well as in maintenance single-agent therapy for advanced ovarian cancer patients in the first-line setting. Furthermore, it has been approved in combination with carboplatin and gemcitabine in platinum-sen-sitive ovarian cancer recurrence. To date, the US Food and Drug Administration (FDA) did not approve it [2]. This lack of consensus EMEA and FDA make reflects concerns about bevacizumab-specific side effects in a palliative situation.

In this chapter, evidence for bevacizumab treatment efficacy in elderly patients will be reviewed, and data on bevacizumab treatment toxicity will be analyzed.

Efficacy

Since 10 years ago, a large amount of data on bevacizumab treatment is accumulat-ing for metastatic cancer patients and especially for colorectal and breast cancers. Indeed, in the late 1990s, phase I clinical trials assessing the safety of this molecule were conducted. It was first approved for metastatic colorectal cancer in 2004, and then it was approved for the treatment of non-squamous non-small cell lung cancer in 2006 and then for metastatic breast cancer in 2008. Several randomized trials, as well as observational cohort studies, showed that the better outcome of the bevaci-zumab combination treatment is similar in elderly patients and in the general study population [3–5].

For ovarian cancers, several phase II and randomized phase III clinical trials have demonstrated an improvement in terms of progression-free survival (PFS) leading to the use of bevacizumab in both frontline chemotherapy and maintenance therapy for advanced disease. Table 7.1 presents the most relevant clinical trials for advanced/recurrent ovarian cancer. Of note, in the large majority of these studies, there were a proportion of patients over the age of 70; however, the characteristics of this specific subpopulation of patients are rarely mentioned. Furthermore, no specific geriatric assessments were published.

In the phase II OCTAVIA trial, the efficacy of the experimental regimen with beva-cizumab (six to eight cycles of bevacizumab with weekly paclitaxel 80 mg/m^2 and carboplatin [AUC6], followed by bevacizumab alone 7.5 mg/kg q3w for up to 1 year) was similar between patients <65 years old and patients ≥65 years old (with a median

Table 7.1 Published clinical trials with bevacizumab for ovarian cancer patients

Clinical trial	Phase	Treatment schema	N	Median age [range]	Responses CR+PR or HR	Median PFS
Cannistra (2007) [6]	II	Bev monotherapy	44	59.5 [31–87]	16 %	4.4 months
Burger (2007) [7]	II	Bev monotherapy	62	57 [18–79]	21 %	4.7 months
Garcia (2008) [8]	II	Bev + daily oral cyclophosphamide	70	60 [31–83]	24 %	7.2 months
Kudoh (2011) [9]	II	Bev + weekly PLD	30	55 [34–69]	33 %	6 months
Asmane (2011)	II	BEV + CT	43	52 [34–77]	40 %	4 months
OCTAVIA (2013) [10]	II	Bev + carboplatin AUC=6 + Weekly paclitaxel	189	55 [24–79]	85 %	23.7 months
GOG0218 (2011) [11]	III	Carboplatin AUC=5 + Paclitaxel q3w ± Bev (± Maintenance Bev)	1873	60 [25–86]	aHR=0.72 95 % CI [0.62–0.82] $p<0.001$	10.3 months versus 14.1 months
ICON7 (2011) [12]	III	Carboplatin AUC=5 + Paclitaxel q3w ± Bev With maintenance	1528	57 [18–82]	HR=0.81 95 % CI [0.70–0.94] $p=0.0041$	17.3 months versus 19.0 months
OCEANS (2012) [13]	III	Carboplatin AUC=4 + Gemcitabine d1d8 ± Bev	484	60 [28–87]	HR=0.48 95 % CI [0.39–0.60] $p<0.001$	8.4 months versus 12.4 months
AURELIA (2014) [14]	III	Paclitaxel or topotecan or PLD ± Bev	361	61 [25–84]	HR=0.48 95 % CI [0.38–0.60] $p<0.001$	3.4 months versus 6.7 months

PFS progression-free survival, *CR* complete response, *PR* partial response, *Bev* bevacizumab, *PLD* PEGylated liposomal doxorubicin
aWhen comparing the chemo + Bev combination followed by maintenance Bev versus chemo alone

PFS of 23.7 and 20.5 months for patients <65 years old and patients ≥65 years old, respectively) [10]. In the two large phase III trials evaluating bevacizumab as first-line therapy in combination with chemotherapy and as maintenance therapy in previously untreated ovarian cancer patients (GOG0218 and ICON7), the PFS of older patients was prolonged with the combination therapy followed by bevacizumab maintenance (versus chemotherapy alone) [11, 12]. In GOG0218, > 300 patients (17 % of the study population) were 70 years old or older (1.7 % were more than 80 years old). In terms of histological profile, elderly patients reported more primary peritoneal disease compared to patients less than 60 (NS). There was a significant improvement in terms of PFS with HR=0.68 for the experimental arm with the maintenance therapy compared to the control arm (chemotherapy alone) [11]. The subgroup analysis of PFS by treatment arm and age reported a similar effect whatever is the age class for patients receiving bevacizumab compared to placebo. HR is 0.81, 0.76, and 0.79 for age class less than 60, 60–69, and 70 or older, respectively, in the bevacizumab arm compared to placebo. There is no detrimental effect also in terms of overall survival using bevacizumab also in the group of patients of 70 years old and more (HR 0.99) compared to placebo. However, age and performance status remain prognostic factors for overall survival in this clinical trial. In the ICON7 trial, 150 patients (10 % of the study population) were 70 years old or older. There was a nonsignificant improvement in terms of progression-free survival, with HR=0.82 [0.51–1.30] [12].

In the OCEAN trial and the AURELIA trial, bevacizumab was evaluated in the relapsed setting. In the OCEAN trial, patients with platinum-sensitive recurrence received carboplatin plus gemcitabine chemotherapy ± bevacizumab followed by maintenance therapy with either bevacizumab or placebo; 178 patients (37 % of the study population) were 65 years old or older. The magnitude of benefit obtained in the bevacizumab arm (compared to the chemotherapy alone arm) was similar between the group of patients <65 years old and the group of patients ≥65 years old (HR=0.47 [0.36–0.62] and 0.50 [0.34–0.72], respectively) [13]. In the AURELIA trial, patients with platinum-resistant recurrent ovarian cancer received single-agent chemotherapy ± bevacizumab; 133 patients (37 % of the study population) were 65 years old or older. The median PFS was significantly improved with chemotherapy plus bevacizumab (versus chemotherapy alone); however, the subgroup analysis by age did not show a statistically significant improvement when comparing the two treatment arms (HR=0.82 [0.61–1.10] for patients <65 years old and HR=0.95 [0.62–1.46] for patients ≥65 years old) [14].

Taken together, these data showed that the benefit from adding bevacizumab treatment to standard chemotherapy as observed in the general population may be also applied to the subpopulation of patients aged over 65 years. Age per se is not an absolute contraindication for bevacizumab.

Toxicity

Specific antiangiogenic agent-related side effects are well known (e.g., hypertension, proteinuria, bleeding, and wound healing complications). Two major phase II clinical trials in ovarian cancer patients have tested the single-agent bevacizumab treatment in patients with recurrent disease. In the first trial, sponsored and monitored by Genentech, Inc. (South San Francisco, CA), the study was stopped after 44 patients' enrollment due to a higher than expected incidence of gastrointestinal (GI) perforations (5 patients). These GI perforations may be related to the advanced nature of their disease. However, 8 patients discontinued the bevacizumab treatment because of an adverse event; 5 patients presented a grade 4 event, and 3 patients had a grade 5 event (one patient died of myocardial infarction and cerebrovascular ischemia, one of intestinal perforation, and one of convulsion and hypertensive encephalopathy). Furthermore, bevacizumab-associated grade 3/4 hypertension, proteinuria, bleeding, venous thromboembolic events, arterial thromboembolic events, wound healing complications, and congestive heart failure were also reported [6]. These results have highlighted the significant risk of the use of bevacizumab in a frail population (e.g., with cardiovascular histories). Nevertheless, four arterial thromboembolic events have been reported in three patients, but all of whom were younger than 65 years.

In the second trial from the GOG group, 62 patients with a median age of 57 years (18–79 years) were enrolled. In contrast with the previous study, no GI perforation was reported, although four patients presented with grade 3/4 GI events. Furthermore, only one patient developed grade 4 proteinuria, and overall side effects were mild and manageable (hypertension grade 3 in 10 %; 2 patients experienced thromboembolic events; no arterial thrombosis was noted) [7].

Hypertension and Proteinuria

In the two large phase III trials GOG0218 and ICON7, bevacizumab treatment was associated with an increase in hypertension of grade 2 or higher (23 % with maintenance bevacizumab versus 7 % with standard therapy in the GOG0218 trial; 18 % with bevacizumab versus 2 % with standard therapy in the ICON7 trial). Clinical management of this hypertension may require standard treatments such as angiotensin-converting enzyme inhibitors [15]. The common occurrence of both hypertension and proteinuria reflect the importance of VEGF in physiological renal function. Although there was no grade 3 proteinuria in the OCTAVIA study (grade 2 in 4 % of patients), the incidence of grade 3 or higher proteinuria in the GOG0218 and ICON7 trials ranged from 0.4 % to 1.6 %. Usually, proteinuria resolves spontaneously at the end of the antiangiogenic treatment.

Thromboembolic Events

Data from 10 randomized trials with cancer patients (other than ovarian) treated with bevacizumab have been pooled to show no statistically significant increase in the incidence of venous thromboembolic events [16]. This has been confirmed in the trials assessing bevacizumab treatment for ovarian cancer patients [10–14].

As previously mentioned, arterial thromboembolic events have been reported in the first phase II study, but for patients younger than 65 years. However, it has been showed that patients with colorectal cancer >65 years old treated with bevacizumab have an increased risk of arterial thromboembolic events compared to younger patients [17]. In the ICON7 trial, 20 patients (3 %) have presented grade 3 or higher arterial thromboembolic events (versus 1 % in the control arm) [12]. In the AURELIA trial, 2 % of patients have presented grade 3 or higher arterial thromboembolic events (versus 0 in the control arm) [14].

Congestive Heart Failure

Since significant increases in the risk of congestive heart failure have been reported for previous studies with metastatic cancer patients treated with bevacizumab [18], patients with mild to serious cardiac conditions have been excluded from the antiangiogenic clinical trials for ovarian cancers.

Wound Healing Complications

Grade 3 or higher wound healing complications have been reported in every bevacizumab clinical trial for ovarian cancer patients (3.6 %, 1 %, and 0.8 % in the GOG0218, ICON7, and OCEAN trials, respectively) [11–13]. This incidence of events appears superior compared to control arms. However, patients with nonhealing wound have been excluded from these trials, and a minimal 4-week interval between antiangiogenic exposure and peritoneal surgery was usually required.

Gastrointestinal Perforation

In the ICON7 trial, gastrointestinal perforations occurred in 10 patients in the bevacizumab arm versus 3 patients in the control arm [11]. A recent analysis of the 1873 patients enrolled onto the GOG0218 trial showed that previous histories of inflammatory bowel disease and bowel resections (small bowel or large bowel) are independently correlated with the incidence of GI perforation. In this study, the rate of GI adverse events was 3.4 % in each bevacizumab treatment group (odds ratio of 2.15 when the group of patients treated with chemotherapy plus bevacizumab were compared to the group of patients treated with chemotherapy alone) [19]. According to the authors, these data suggests that impairment of healing at sites of GI injury due to bevacizumab treatment is a possible mechanism explaining the increased rate of GI perforation for ovarian cancer patients treated with bevacizumab. It remains that tumor infiltration of the mesentery, blood flow interruption, bowel obstruction, and previous abdominal surgery are very common in ovarian cancer patients, and assessment of GI wall impairment (especially anastomotic dehiscence) remains difficult in the routine clinic. The question of the age of the patient as a risk factor for GI perforation remains unclear. In a retrospective review of 160 patients with recurrent ovarian carcinoma who had been treated with bevacizumab, 6 cases of GI perforations were reported. The median age of these patients was 69 years (range,

48–83) (versus 61 years, range 21–88, in the entire cohort). Four patients were older than 65 years old (66, 73, 75, and 85 years old), and all of them have died within the first 2 months following the diagnosis of GI perforation [20].

Management in the Clinical Practice

Taken together, these data are consistent with an excess of GI and arterial severe adverse events for elderly patients, especially if those patients who present with more advanced disease. Indeed, in the first phase II trial [6], patients presented platinum-resistant cancers and had received >2 previous chemotherapy. Their performance status was poorer (59 % of PS=0 and 41 % of PS=1 in the Cannistra's trial versus 73 % of PS=0 and 17 % of PS=1 in the Burger's trial). The study was stopped due to a higher than expected severe adverse events. Consequently, one can argue that appropriate selection of patients should reduce the risk of GI and vascular adverse events related to bevacizumab treatment.

Ordering bevacizumab for ovarian cancer patients aged >70 years is usually based only on the physicians' experience. No validated score may help to discuss this therapeutic option in this specific population. Since older patients included in clinical trials do not represent the general elderly population, it remains unknown if advanced age by itself may be a risk factor for the development of bevacizumab-induced vascular/GI adverse events. Exclusion criteria of the majority of clinical trials using antiangiogenic agents included history of bleeding or thrombosis, strokes, significant cardiac events (ischemic or congestive heart failure), and uncontrolled hypertension. Thus, antiangiogenic agents should not be administered or may be administered with a lot of caution in patients with mild/severe cardiovascular conditions.

Regarding the risk of GI perforation, there is no recommendation to avoid antiangiogenic agent due to age, and previous histories of injuries on the GI tract must prevail in the discussion to prescribe bevacizumab treatment. In the AURELIA trial, patients were excluded if they had presented history of bowel obstruction/abdominal fistula or if they had clinical evidence of recto-sigmoid involvement; in this study, the rate of GI perforation was low [14].

In our routine clinic, we have determined factors associated with the onset of fistulas and GI perforations. It appeared that prior history of multiple (>2) surgical procedures, pelvic radiation therapy, and hyperthermic intraperitoneal chemotherapy procedure were significantly associated with an increased risk of fistula and GI perforations for ovarian cancer patients treated with bevacizumab plus microtubule-targeting agents [21].

Most importantly, it has been persistently reported that chemotherapy-related side effects are higher in patients receiving chemotherapy plus bevacizumab than in those receiving either treatment alone. In the GOG0218, most adverse events were reported during the chemotherapy phase rather than during the bevacizumab maintenance phase. All but one GI perforation occurred during the chemotherapy courses [11]. Similarly, in the OCTAVIA trial, all reported GI perforation appeared during the concurrent chemotherapy plus bevacizumab treatment (no GI perforation was noted during the single-agent bevacizumab phase) [10]. Consequently, the use of chemotherapy plus bevacizumab combination should always be prescribed with caution in elderly patients with peritoneal carcinomatosis, meaning that the benefit/risk ratio should be regularly reassessed.

Conclusion

As a clinician's experience of bevacizumab treatment has increased over time, the selection of older patients eligible for antiangiogenic agents can be better achieved. Indeed, in a recent study, specifically designed for elderly patients (median age of 74 years) with metastatic colorectal cancers ($n=44$), most bevacizumab-related severe adverse events were limited to grade 1/2 (two patients had grade 3 hypertension, and one patient experienced grade 3 GI perforation) [22]. Age by itself should not be used as a strict limit for the use of antiangiogenic agents. Thus, in a pooled analysis of four randomized studies with bevacizumab for colorectal cancer patients, it appears that there was no major increase in terms of adverse events for patients aged over 75 years compared to patients <75 years old [3]. Nevertheless, contraindications to the bevacizumab must be respected. For instance, in a recent population-based analysis aimed to determine the predictors of bevacizumab use in elderly patients with metastatic colon, lung, and breast cancers, it has been showed that the drug was used commonly in patients who present contraindications to the drug (one third of patients) [23]. Consequently, complications resulting from bevacizumab treatment were significantly higher than have been reported in randomized clinical trials.

Hypertension and proteinuria were the only bevacizumab-related SAEs reported more frequently in older than in younger patients (the relationship between presence or severity of baseline hypertension and the severity of bevacizumab-induced hypertension is uncertain). In the clinical trials dedicated to bevacizumab in ovarian cancer, no differences in AEs leading to discontinuation or death were reported specifically in this population. We are waiting for subgroup analyses concerning other antiangiogenics (as pazopanib, nintedanib, cediranib) for this population of elderly ovarian cancer. Today, antiangiogenic agents may be prescribed for ovarian cancer patients irrespective of age, with a careful benefit/risk ratio evaluation and a systematic monitoring for potential adverse events.

References

1. Horowitz JR, Rivard A, van der Zee R, et al. Vascular endothelial growth factor/vascular permeability factor produces nitric oxide-dependent hypotension. Evidence for a maintenance role in quiescent adult endothelium. Arterioscler Thromb Vasc Biol. 1997;17:2793–800.
2. Liu JF, Cannistra SA. Emerging role for bevacizumab in combination with chemotherapy for patients with platinum-resistant ovarian cancer. J Clin Oncol. 2014;32:1287–9.
3. Cassidy J, Saltz LB, Giantonio BJ, et al. Effect of bevacizumab in older patients with metastatic colorectal cancer: pooled analysis of four randomized studies. J Cancer Res Clin Oncol. 2010;136:737–43.
4. Price TJ, Zannino D, Wilson K, et al. Bevacizumab is equally effective and no more toxic in elderly patients with advanced colorectal cancer: a subgroup analysis from the AGITG MAX

trial: an international randomised controlled trial of capecitabine, bevacizumab and mitomycin C. Ann Oncol. 2012;23:1531–6.

5. Biganzoli L, di Vincenzo E, Jiang Z, et al. First-line bevacizumab-containing therapy for breast cancer: results in patients aged ≥70 years treated in the ATHENA study. Ann Oncol. 2012;23:111–8.

6. Cannistra SA, Matulonis UA, Penson RT, et al. Phase II study of bevacizumab in patients with platinum-resistant ovarian cancer or peritoneal serous cancer. J Clin Oncol. 2007;25:5180–6.

7. Burger RA, Sill MW, Monk BJ, et al. Phase II trial of bevacizumab in persistent or recurrent epithelial ovarian cancer or primary peritoneal cancer: a Gynecologic Oncology Group Study. J Clin Oncol. 2007;25:5165–71.

8. Garcia AA, Hirte H, Fleming G, et al. Phase II clinical trial of bevacizumab and low-dose metronomic oral cyclophosphamide in recurrent ovarian cancer: a trial of the California, Chicago, and Princess Margaret Hospital phase II consortia. J Clin Oncol. 2008;26:76–82.

9. Kudoh K, Takano M, Kouta H, et al. Effects of bevacizumab and pegylated liposomal doxorubicin for the patients with recurrent or refractory ovarian cancers. Gynecol Oncol. 2011;122:233–7.

10. Gonzalez-Martin A, Gladieff L, Tholander B, OCTAVIA Investigators, et al. Efficacy and safety results from OCTAVIA, a single-arm phase II study evaluating front-line bevacizumab, carboplatin and weekly paclitaxel for ovarian cancer. Eur J Cancer. 2013;49:3831–8.

11. Burger RA, Brady MF, Bookman MA, et al. Incorporation of bevacizumab in the primary treatment of ovarian cancer. N Engl J Med. 2011;365:2473–83.

12. Perren TJ, Swart AM, Pfisterer J, et al. A phase 3 trial of bevacizumab in ovarian cancer. N Engl J Med. 2011;365:2484–96.

13. Aghajanian C, Blank SV, Goff BA, et al. OCEANS: a randomized, double-blind, placebo-controlled phase III trial of chemotherapy with or without bevacizumab in patients with platinum-sensitive recurrent epithelial ovarian, primary peritoneal, or fallopian tube cancer. J Clin Oncol. 2012;30:2039–45.

14. Pujade-Lauraine E, Hilpert F, Weber B, et al. Bevacizumab combined with chemotherapy for platinum-resistant recurrent ovarian cancer: the AURELIA open-label randomized phase III trial. J Clin Oncol. 2014;32:1302–8.

15. Dincer M, Altundag K. Angiotensin-converting enzyme inhibitors for bevacizumab-induced hypertension. Ann Pharmacother. 2006;40:2278–9.

16. Hurwitz HI, Saltz LB, van Cutsem E, et al. Venous thromboembolic events with chemotherapy plus bevacizumab: a pooled analysis of patients in randomized phase II and III studies. J Clin Oncol. 2011;29:1757–64.

17. Scappaticci FA, Skillings JR, Holden SN, et al. Arterial thromboembolic events in patients with metastatic carcinoma treated with chemotherapy and bevacizumab. J Natl Cancer Inst. 2007;99:1232–9.

18. Choueiri TK, Mayer EL, Je Y, et al. Congestive heart failure risk in patients with breast cancer treated with bevacizumab. J Clin Oncol. 2011;29:632–8.

19. Burger RA, Brady MF, Bookman MA, et al. Risk factors for GI adverse events in a phase III randomized trial of Bevacizumab in first-line therapy of advanced ovarian cancer: a Gynecologic Oncology Group Study. J Clin Oncol. 2014;32:1210–7.

20. Diaz JP, Tew WP, Zivanovic O, et al. Incidence and management of bevacizumab-associated gastrointestinal perforations in patients with recurrent ovarian carcinoma. Gynecol Oncol. 2010;116:335–9.

21. Asmane I, Kurtz JE, Bajard A, et al. Bevacizumab plus microtubule targeting agents in heavily pre-treated ovarian cancer patients: a retrospective study. Bull Cancer. 2011;98:80–9.

22. Rosati G, Avallone A, Aprile G, et al. XELOX and bevacizumab followed by single-agent bevacizumab as maintenance therapy as first-line treatment in elderly patients with advanced colorectal cancer: the boxe study. Cancer Chemother Pharmacol. 2013;71:257–64.

23. Hershman DL, Wright JD, Lim E, et al. Contraindicated use of bevacizumab and toxicity in elderly patients with cancer. J Clin Oncol. 2013;31:3592–9.

How to Design Clinical Trials?

8

Sandro Pignata, Sabrina Chiara Cecere, and Rosa Tambaro

Contents

Introduction

Ovarian cancer (OC) is the leading cause of mortality among patients with gynecologic malignancies [1]. More than half of all OC occurs in women older than 65 [1, 2]. The vast majority of women with ovarian cancer present with advanced stages, and curative treatment requires both aggressive surgery and chemotherapy. This approach has resulted in an improvement of the survival rates in the general population over the last decades with a median survival exceeding 50 months in

S. Pignata (✉) • S.C. Cecere • R. Tambaro
Dipartimento Uro-Ginecologico, Istituto Nazionale Tumori "Fondazione G Pascale" – IRCCS, Naples, Italy
e-mail: s.pignata@istitutotumori.na.it

© Springer International Publishing Switzerland 2016
G. Freyer (ed.), *Ovarian Cancer in Elderly Patients*,
DOI 10.1007/978-3-319-23588-2_8

most published series; the improvement is not present in the elderly population [3, 4].

Although older adults account for the majority of cancer incidence and mortality, few clinical trials have focused on this patient population [5]. Several groups reported at least a twofold increase risk of death in women older than age 65 years [6, 7]. Various theories have been proposed to account for this survival disparity in older women, including: (1) more aggressive cancer with advanced age; (2) inherent resistance to chemotherapy; (3) individual patient factors, such as multiple concurrent medical problems; and (4) physician and healthcare biases toward the elderly, which lead to inadequate surgery, less than optimal chemotherapy, and poor enrollment in clinical trials [8]. Ovarian cancer patients aged ≥70 years do frequently not receive optimal multimodal therapy despite treatment in specialized cancer centers, and their outcome is significantly impaired despite no consistent prognostic effect of age [9].

Undertreatment is the main determinant of the worse prognosis in elderly ovarian cancer patients. Debulking surgery with the intent of complete tumor resection is frequently feasible, even in advanced disease stages [10] However, cytoreduction often requires radical surgical steps like bowel resection, upper abdominal surgery or pelvic surgery, as well as para-aortic lymphadenectomy. In this context, a major concern of surgeons is the fear of a higher complication and mortality rate. According to SEER Cancer Statistic review, age remains the most predictive factor for suboptimal surgical management [11].

The same occurs for chemotherapy. Elderly patients are less frequently treated with an adequate medical treatment. Thus, it is clear that there is a need for trials including elderly patients to define guidelines and reduce undertreatment.

An important point of debate is related to the end points to be chosen in clinical trials in elderly patients.

Studies specifically concentrating on the distinct needs and expectations of elderly patients are highly desirable. These trials should also consider that apart from effects on overall survival and progression-free survival, other goals may be important for elderly patients. While in general oncology, well-established end points for clinical research exist, it may not be as relevant to the older cancer population because of competing risks of death and potentially increased impact of therapy on global functioning and quality of life.

Some authors have claimed that older adult patients with incurable disease may prefer QoL to the extension of lifetime, especially if treatment also has an impact on their functional capacity and ability to carry out daily tasks, their cognitive function, their social situation/capability to stay at home, or their caregiving abilities [12].

Therefore, there is a need for delineation of relevant clinical end points for older individuals, which can then be uniformly incorporated into future clinical trials [13, 14].

Which Elderly Patients Should Be Included in Clinical Trials?

The growing worldwide population of older adults has been underrepresented in clinical trials that set the standards for oncology care. In the Southwest Oncology Group (SWOG) analysis of data on 16,396 patients enrolled in 164 trials during the

1990s, patients with OC older than 65 accounted for only 30 % of all included patients [15]. Similarly, in a recent Surveillance, Epidemiology, and End Results (SEER) survey, only 9 % of patients with cancer older than 75 were included in clinical trials of new therapies [16]. Although in the last decade improvement in the enrollment of older adults in clinical trials has occurred, the representation of older adults on trials is still far from ideal, and the enrollment fraction of patients 75 and older in clinical trials (i.e., the number enrolled divided by estimated cancer cases) worsens with increasing age. Perhaps the most concerning statistics is that older adults are underrepresented in registration trials of new drugs approved by regulatory authorities, despite the FDA's recommendation to include older adults in clinical trials [16]. As a result, the standard drug dosing and expected side effect profile is primarily derived from a younger cohort of patients.

Two possible strategies may be adopted: to increase the number of elderly patients in conventional trials for adult or to design trials specific for elderly people who are not candidates for conventional therapies. However, how can we define the patients that can enter and those not suitable for conventional clinical trials?

Chronological age is no longer a valid exclusion criterion, and the majority of adult cooperative group clinical trials no longer specify an upper age limit. In fact, it is believed that the clinical applicability of the results of a cancer treatment trial depends largely on whether the study participants are representative of the population of interest [17]. Hence, to ensure that clinical trial results are generalizable to older patients, trials should include them in numbers proportional to their distribution among the cancer population.

However, the majority of cancer trials prohibit participation of people with hematologic, hepatic, renal, or cardiac abnormalities. Exclusions on the basis of hypertension, cardiac disease, hematologic, or pulmonary function abnormalities resulted in 8.6 %, 5.3 %, 14.1 %, and 9.3 % lower enrollment of older patients, respectively, in National Cancer Institute (NCI) trials from 1997 to 2000 [18]. Aging is associated with several physiologic changes in organ function that could alter drug pharmacokinetics and have an impact on cytotoxic chemotherapy tolerability and toxicity [19]. Renal function, as indicated by the glomerular filtration rate, is reduced with age [20]. Bone marrow reserves diminish with increasing age, and myelotoxicity can be substantially increased [21].

Multiple comorbid diseases are common in elderly cancer patients. The overall burden of comorbidities has a negative impact on patient's survival [22, 23] and on the patient's ability to tolerate treatment or may be a contraindication for cancer treatment (e.g., trastuzumab in patients with congestive heart failure).

In an observational study of 17,712 patients with a new primary diagnosis of cancer, survival was found to be inversely related to age, and comorbid medical conditions had an impact on survival independent of cancer stage [23].

Thus, the only way to encourage the participation of elderly people in conventional clinical trials would be to clearly define in the protocol, when there is no clear contraindication, dose adjustment, and titration strategies for patients with mild functional abnormalities related to comorbidities. In fact comorbidity conditions and toxicity are considered by physicians as the most frequently potential barriers to trial enrollment [18, 24]. Other factors that physicians consider as a barrier to enrollment are the lack of support for the older patient to manage side effects at home, transportation needs in case of toxicity, or simply that life expectancy of some patients is too short to justify participation in clinical trials [18, 25].

However, even in the case where the protocol clearly defines rules to encourage the participation of elderly people, including wider inclusion criteria and defining clear dose adjustment rules according to comorbidities, there is a proportion of aged patients that we do not feel to be safely included in conventional trials and that in our view should be included in dedicated elderly trials.

In other words these patients are vulnerable or fragile and at serious risk of excess toxicity from surgery or standard medical treatments.

Frailty is defined as a state of decreased physiological reserve and increased susceptibility to suffer disability in response to stressors [26–28]. How frailty is measured varies between a physical assessment and a more physiological assessment. Makary and colleagues used a validated scoring system of physical frailty in a prospective study of patients older than 65 presenting for elective surgery. The frailty score was based on five domains, which included weight loss, weakness, exhaustion, low physical activity, and slowed walking speed [26]. This frailty score was then compared with more conventional preoperative assessments such as the ASA score, Lee's revised cardiac index, and Eagle score. Frailty was found to correlate with postoperative complications with an adjusted odds ratio of 1.78–2.13 for intermediately frail patients and 2.48–3.15 in frail patients. Frailty was also correlated with increased length of stay (65–89 % longer stays for frail patients) and nontraditional discharge [28]. Other investigators have looked at physiological frailty as a predictor of outcome in preoperative patients. Domains studied included comorbidity, function, nutrition, cognition, geriatric syndrome assessment, and extrinsic frailty (social support) [28]. Using this assessment of frailty, following factors found were associated most closely with 6-month mortality: cognitive dysfunction, lower albumin, having fallen in the previous 6 months, lower hematocrit, functional dependence, and increased comorbidities. Having four or more of these markers predicted 6-month mortality with a sensitivity of 86 % [28]. Although older adults have been identified as being vulnerable to side effects from cancer therapy, few oncology studies to date have specifically incorporated baseline metrics for measuring health conditions other than functional status (Eastern Cooperative Oncology Group [ECOG] or Karnofsky performance status [PS]) to identify individuals most at risk. Until recently, a consistent definition of frailty remained elusive.

Thus, the clear definition in the protocol of the type of elderly people that are enrolled is the first mandatory step when designing a clinical trial in this setting.

Tools to Better Define Elderly Cancer Patients Included in Either Conventional or Elderly Specific Clinical Trials

The cutoff point at which an adult is considered "old" has not been well defined. Traditionally, a chronological landmark has been considered the age of 70. After this age, it is reported an increased incidence of age-related physiological changes, risk factor for altered pharmacokinetics and pharmacodynamics, potentially leading to increased treatment-related toxicity [29].

However, this cutoff is arbitrary. Aging is a highly individualized process, and all changes involved in this process cannot be predicted solely on the basis of chronological age. Aging has been defined as a loss of "entropy and fractality" [30]. Loss of "entropy" implies a progressive reduction in an individual's functional reserve, whereas loss of "fractality" implies a progressive reduction in the ability to coordinate different activity and negotiate the environment.

Trials should be designed to capture functional reserve and ability of elderly patients. Furthermore, coexisting medical problems also led to significant use of medication; polypharmacy has been reported as a significant factor which contributes to increased chemotherapy toxicity.

Older adults may be particularly susceptible to polypharmacy, given the increased number of comorbidities in this population. Polypharmacy raises the likelihood of adverse drug reactions in older cancer patients and has been associated with increased mortality [31].

A strict assessment of comorbidities and polypharmacy in clinical trials is required because it will determine the patients' life expectancy and clarify the generalizability of the results of the trial. CRF must be clearly designed to capture this scenario.

Comprehensive Geriatric Assessment in Clinical Trials

In clinical practice, the major issue of the older population is heterogeneity. Some older patients will tolerate chemotherapy or surgery as well as their younger counterparts, while others will experience severe toxicity, requiring treatment reduction, treatment delay, or permanent discontinuation. Thus, a major issue confronted by oncologists treating older cancer patients is how to effectively select patients suitable for standard or attenuated therapy. This is mainly relevant for treatments such as classical chemotherapy and high risk surgery, which can have severe potential impact on functionality, quality of life (morbidity), and even potentially life-threatening toxicity (iatrogenic mortality).

Comprehensive geriatric assessment (CGA) is an approach developed and used by the geriatricians to set up an individualized and proactive care plan. It evaluates the patients' global and functional status, in order to improve treatment decisions and outcomes. The definition of CGA according to the consensus conference, supported by the National Institute of Aging in 1989, states the following: *CGA is a multidimensional, interdisciplinary patient evaluation that leads to the identification of patient's problems.*

CGA assesses the presence of comorbidities, mental status and emotional conditions, social support, the nutritional status of the elderly patient, polypharmacy, and the presence or absence of geriatric syndromes [32, 33]. CGA is useful for detecting reversible factors that interfere with treatment (inadequate social support, malnutrition, reversible comorbidity, etc.); estimating the risk for mortality according to the functional state of the patient, the degree of comorbidity (e.g., depression and anemia are associated with increased mortality), and the presence of geriatric syndromes; and estimating tolerance to chemotherapy, which is lower in patients with functional dependency, comorbidity, malnutrition, and/or anemia [34].

It has been shown that CGA has a better relevance and accuracy in the cancer patient than a simple clinical evaluation, such as PS assessment [35].

Data concerning CGA and its ability to detect unknown health problems in elderly cancer population are consistent and promote its use in clinical practice and in clinical trials including elderly patients. A pilot study assessed the ability of repeated CGAs to detect undiagnosed or undertreated problems in breast cancer patients (median age 79): An average of six unaddressed/underaddressed problems/patients were detected at baseline, and three new problems occurred over the following months [36].

The prognostic and predictive role of CGA has been investigated in multiple studies. Winkelmann and colleagues [37] reported a prospective trial with 143 patients newly diagnosed with malignant lymphoma who were evaluated by CGA including ADL, IADL, and comorbidities. In a Cox regression analysis, IADL (hazard ratio [HR] 2.1; 95 % confidence interval [CI] 1.1–3.9) and comorbidity (HR 1.9; 95 % CI 0.9–3.9) were independent and most strongly associated with survival time.

CGA has been also used in ovarian cancer trials. In the GINECO "carboplatin-cyclophosphamide" study, three factors seemed to have a poor prognostic value, of which two emerged from the CGA: symptoms of depression and more than six comedications taken daily, along with FIGO stage IV [38]. In the final analysis done pooling two GINECO studies (155 patients included), symptoms of depression had an independent poor prognostic value (hazard ratio=5.11, PG 0.001), as well as FIGO stage IV, paclitaxel use, and lymphopenia at study entry [39].

Furthermore, in the Freyer et al. experience, CGA was also promising in enlightening health parameters linked to severe treatment-related toxicity. In their prospective analysis conducted over a 12-year interval, 83 patients aged 70 years and older with advanced ovarian carcinoma who were treated with carboplatin and paclitaxel were included. A geriatric assessment was performed prior to the initiation of therapy. Several elements of the geriatric assessment predicted the occurrence of severe toxicity with chemotherapy, including depression ($P \leq .003$) and intake of six or more medications per day ($P \leq .043$) [38].

A recent review evaluating the role of CGA in 411 controlled trials shows a diversity of affected domains correlating with the different end points. Nutritional status, functionality, and comorbidity were most often associated with worse outcome and severe toxicity caused by chemotherapy. In addition geriatric assessment revealed unknown geriatric problems in more than 50 % of oncogeriatric patients, and 21–53 % of chemotherapy regimens were modified based on CGA [40].

Recently, two models predicting the risk of severe side effects from chemotherapy in older patients have been proposed: The Chemotherapy Risk Assessment Scale for High-Age Patients (CRASH) score [41] and the Cancer and Aging Research Group score [42] validated in some studies, but not routinely integrated in CGA.

The CGA approach allows the discrimination of patients into three broad categories: (a) fit elderly patients who do not have any serious comorbidity and no dependence (fit patients), (b) frail patients with significant dependency and comorbidities, and finally (c) patients with some IADL dependency with or without severe comorbidity (vulnerable patients). Patients in the first group are good candidates for almost every form of cancer treatment as they tolerate anticancer treatment as well as their younger counterparts with similar outcomes in terms of survival [43]. These patients can be included in conventional clinical trials increasing the generalizability of the results.

Patients of the second group are usually offered only best supportive care or only single-agent palliative chemotherapy, while for the third category of patients, which is the biggest, individualized approaches are recommended [44]. The two latter categories are those where specific clinical trials should be designed.

The literature needs information from all the three categories of elderly patients, but it is very important that when reporting results or designing trial this distinction is made clear.

Besides its prognostic role in medical oncology, preoperative CGA assessment of elderly cancer patients before elective surgery also showed similar effectiveness in evaluating oncogeriatric fitness for surgery and predicting perioperative complications in elderly patients and this may be of particular importance in ovarian cancer. At the 2011 American Society of Clinical Oncology Annual Meeting, Basso and colleagues [45] presented the results of a prospective cohort of older cancer patients who received a multidimensional geriatric assessment. Patients who were fit according to Balducci criteria had a 2-year survival of 83 %, those who were vulnerable 70 %, and those who were frail 60 %.

A validated instrument for presurgical assessment of the elderly or patients with OC who have performance status challenges does not yet exist. The PACE (Preoperative Assessment of Cancer in the Elderly) tool was developed to combine elements of the CGA with surgical risk tools. Instruments included in the PACE are a mini-mental state inventory, activities of daily living (ADLs), instrumental activities of daily living (IADLs), geriatric depression scale (GDS), brief fatigue inventory (BFI), ECOG performance status (PS), ASA and Satariano's index of comorbidities. This tool has been studied prospectively among 460 patients undergoing surgery for breast cancer, gastrointestinal cancer, genitourinary cancer, and others. Researchers found no significant association of age with postoperative complications. IADL, moderate to severe BFI, and abnormal PS were most predictive of 30 days morbidity; ADL, IADL, and PS were associated with extended hospital stay [46, 47]. However, even if this approach was able to predict the risk of both postsurgical complications and extended hospital stay, predictive accuracy of this approach needs to be further validated in future studies.

Although CGA clearly reveals extra information, and the International Society of Geriatric Oncology (SIOG) recommends a CGA-based approach to elderly cancer patients, full geriatric assessment of every patient older than 65 years remains a challenge for a busy oncological department but may be highly recommendable for clinical trials including elderly patients.

Due to the complexity of CGA, some authors used simple and short screening questionnaires. Two examples of shorter surveys include the Cancer and Aging Research Group (CARG) Geriatric Assessment and Toxicity Score and The Geriatric Vulnerability Score (GVS). CARG-GA is a feasible assessment (mean time to completion is 27 min, mostly self-administered), and the shorter toxicity score predicted grade 3–5 chemotherapy toxicity [42].

In the GINECO phase II study, Freyer et al. identified six prognostic factors of poorer survival: low albumin (<35 g/L), low ADL score (<6), low IADL score (<25), lymphopenia (<1G/L), and a high HADS score (>14). Based on these predictive factors, the authors developed a scoring system. The Geriatric Vulnerability Score (GVS) was validated on a bootstrap analysis to predict survival, both in the EOC 2 and EOC 3 studies [48]. With a cutoff of three, the number of factors identified two groups of patients with different prognostic outcomes and tolerance to chemotherapy. Indeed, patients with a GVS score ≥ 3 had a worse OS (11.5 months vs. 21.7 months, respectively; HR, 2.94; $p < 10$–4); experienced a lower rate of chemotherapy completion (65 % compared with 82 %, respectively; OR = 0.41; $p = 0.04$); a higher incidence of adverse events (53 % vs. 29 %; OR = 2.8; $p = 0.009$); and higher incidence of unplanned hospitalization (53 % vs. 30 %; OR = 2.6; $p = 0.02$). The use of GVS score appears helpful in selecting those at greatest risk; validation studies with larger cohorts are needed [49].

In conclusion, there is no unique model of CGA in oncogeriatrics. Different models have been published, but each of them has been applied interchangeably to several types of cancer and tumoral stages. Actually, there is sufficient evidence indicating that such an assessment should be carried out at least in clinical trials. According to the SIOG education committee guidelines, a screening tool can be used initially for risk detection. If the screening indicates the presence of a geriatric risk profile, a CGA should be performed and geriatric interventions performed.

The screening tools consist of a combination of clinical tests in different health domains in order to find a sensitive, specific, and simple instrument. Several shorter screening tools have been tested, the most frequently used are Vulnerable Elders Survey (VES-13) [50], Flemish version of the Triage Risk Screening Tool, the Groningen Frailty Indicator (GFI) [51], and the G8 instrument [52].

This "two-step" approach has been recommended in the guidelines of the National Comprehensive Cancer Network (NCCN), the European Organisation for Research and Treatment of Cancer (EORTC), and the International Society of Geriatric Oncology (SIOG) [53] and can be recommendable for conventional clinical trials including elderly patients.

Traditional and Specific End Points for Clinical Trials for Older Patient with Cancer

Although cancer clinical trials are essential in evaluating the safety and efficacy of novel anticancer agents, only 3 % of newly diagnosed cancer patients participate in clinical trials annually [54]. There are a number of design issues which need to be addressed, particularly pertinent to the older patients. Clinical investigators and bio-statisticians need to develop tools to optimize the data derived from these studies. There are many changes to be made to clinical trials designed on a population of elderly, and many potential areas that may be targeted to optimize recruitment of a proportional number of older patients.

Overall Survival

The inclusion of older patients in clinical trials may lower the reported OS rate as a result of deaths from apparently unrelated causes [55, 56]. The causes of death differ between the elderly and younger patients. Particular care must be taken when overall survival is one of study end points. Many trials demonstrate that, particularly, in cancers that have an indolent course, there is a higher rate of all-cause mortality in older patients versus younger patients [57]. In order to avoid biases related to non-cancer mortality, other objectives related to the elderly patient may be added in the trial design as surrogate end points: progression-free survival, period of time without symptoms, treatment-free intervals, and maintenance of independence are all tools that can be associated to OS when assessing efficacy in elderly patients.

Clinical/Functional Benefit

The efficacy of a treatment in terms of response rate is often included among the primary end points of phase 2 studies. Assessment of clinical benefit has become an important end point, especially in the management of metastatic disease, and some agents, including gemcitabine for pancreatic cancer [58] and mitoxantrone and abiraterone for prostate cancer [59, 60], have been approved for use because of demonstrated clinical benefits.

Elderly women with ovarian cancer often have limited life expectancies and impaired PS being at risk of exclusion from clinical trials. As mentioned before, assessment of vulnerability and fragility purely based on the PS is extremely inadequate in the elderly population. Removing PS from exclusion criteria is one of the possible solutions. On the other hand, every study that includes a population of elderly patients should adopt a universally accepted valuation scale both for defining inclusion/exclusion criteria and for later evaluation of functional changes and clinical benefit associated to the investigated treatment [49, 61]. Functional issues can be an appropriate end point; data collection at the start of the trial should include a form of geriatric assessment specific for the elderly patients with cancer. This assessment can be used to better understand the role that a medical treatment has for that specific category of patients and so to recognize the usefulness of chemotherapy in improving symptoms, prevent functional dependence and functional deterioration in metastatic disease or, on the contrary, in reducing functional abilities in patients under treatment.

Quality of Life (QoL)

The main goal of cancer treatment, particularly in the palliative setting, should be to reduce discomfort related to cancer progression and its related consequences. QoL is a major concern for patient with cancer, and it can be affected by symptoms caused by cancer as well as by treatment-induced toxicity. For many older patients, the goal of cancer-directed treatment is not just how much additional time they can gain but how valuable that time is. Patient's QoL is affected by factors related to the cancer and treatment, as well as the interaction with other diseases. Therefore, the assessment of quality of life in clinical trials is a fundamental end point. However, it remains to be defined how to measure or quantify QoL optimally in elderly women. Traditional QoL tools probably need to be enriched with some items of the comprehensive geriatric assessment, focusing on issues like the ability to fully function in social roles and to participate in daily activities, selecting those that are among the most important to older persons. However, many different forms of QoL/geriatric assessment exist that risk to make complicated comparisons across trials.Many trials in ovarian cancer include the FACT-O questionnaire or the EORTC (European Organisation for Research and Treatment of Cancer) QoL questionnaire C30 that has been recently updated in an elderly specific QoL module (International validation of the EORTC QLQ-ELD14 questionnaire for assessment of health-related quality of life of elderly patients with cancer) [62]. It is important to agree on uniform evaluation of the elderly and to continue international discussion on this topic.

Dose-Limiting Toxicity Issues

Toxicity related to treatment is dependent on the type and dose intensity of the therapy, the type and stage of cancer, the underlying biology of the cancer, and differences in functional reserve of the different organ systems. Platinum-/taxane-based chemotherapy is the cornerstone of therapy in ovarian cancer and may carry a significant toxicity with potential important effects on elderly patient's QoL. The older patient may present different side effects than a younger patient. On the other hand, many conditions that would not be considered normal in a younger population are routinely accepted in older people as a part of so-called "normal" aging. Among these many chronic and debilitating conditions such as chronic pain, insomnia, weakness, fatigue, and anemia are frequently reported by the elderly [63]. In other cases a specific toxicity, as in the case of neurotoxicity, may not be more common in the elderly, although the consequences are likely to become more disabling with advancing age, interfering significantly with daily activities and quality of life [64, 65]. Schedule and formulation changes may also alter the toxicity profile of chemotherapy in the aging population. Organ dysfunction studies may be particularly valuable to define the dose of a drug in both younger and older patients [66]. The common toxicity criteria as currently used may not be adequate to assess adverse events in older patients. For example, assessment of neuropathy should include evaluation of functional decline or falls. The reporting of toxicity should be age specific as well. Most trials only report grade 3/4 toxicity, but grade 2 toxicity in an older patient may have clinical relevance.

In-depth evaluation of dose-dependent toxicities in the older patient and the effects of dose modifications on comorbid conditions and outcomes will enable researchers to build dose-modification strategies into future protocols, thereby enhancing recruitment of older patients. We believe that time should be dedicated when designing a clinical trial to this fundamental topic: toxicity according to comorbidities, toxicity according to predefined dose adjustment, and specific interaction of some toxicities with QoL.

It has been proposed that an appropriate selection [67] of elderly patients may allow their inclusion also in dedicated phase I clinical trials that typically include patients with good PS and normal organ function, differing from what has been done historically.

Polypharmacy Issues

At least 90 % of older patients use at least one medication, and the average is approximately eight medications per patient [68]. Older ambulatory patients use threefold more medications than younger counterparts [69]. Polypharmacy registration may be important to better define pharmacokinetic interactions. Trials in elderly patients should not exclude patients who are taking more of a certain number of drugs, but special attention has to be paid to specific medications that might affect the metabolism of the study drug. Significant drug interactions, particularly those involved in the cytochrome P450 system, are of major concern [70–72].

Discussion

Age is a strong predictor of survival in ovarian cancer and often influences the treatment plan. Elderly patients are commonly not offered participation in clinical research. More elderly patients should be included in conventional clinical trials for adult and specific trials should be designed for patients not considered suitable for conventional trials. In both cases factors that accompany aging, such as comorbidities and polypharmacy, have to be captured. The use of a multidimensional geriatric evaluation has been proposed in order to better select patients at high risk of toxicity with the aim of developing the best therapeutic plan for each individual patient. CGA allows to give the imprinting of the population that is included in a trial with elderly people and makes the results comparable.

Many actions should be made to improve clinical cancer trials for the older adult. First, to limit retrospective evaluations that are biased by selection of patients. In prospective trials with a participation of both young and older patients, an analysis of the possible interaction between age, toxicity, and clinical outcome should be preplanned according to patient comorbidity and function characteristics. QoL assessment is a fundamental end point in elderly patients, but has to be matched with the maintenance of functional ability.

It is highly advised that safety assessment of the treatment should include in details every grade of toxicity, particularly those of grade 2 that can be highly significant in the elderly patient. Trials should be designed with stratification for age at study entry and/or with exclusion criteria related to comorbid conditions, functional status, defined in order to not discriminate older patients. Also, better geriatric assessment with functional evaluation is crucial to differentiate the "normal" older patient from the "frail" or "vulnerable" older patient.

After drugs have been approved at doses applicable to patients with an adequate performance status, other studies should also be designed for frail and vulnerable populations to determine whether lower or titrated doses of these drugs can be given safely and if they are effective in the reduced doses.

Choosing end points for clinical trials in older patient with cancer requires careful reflection on the ultimate goals of therapies. OS is an important end point, but disease-specific survival should also be recorded in trials where older patients with cancer are included, because deaths resulting from other causes occur much more frequently in older population. Specific trials for subgroups of older patients with cancer are needed, with additional end points such as QoL ability and functional items that in this setting may be as important as duration of life.

To improve treatment guidelines, more clinical trials specifically designed for older patients should be implemented. In addition, enhanced cooperation focused on this topic between geriatricians, medical oncologists, and gynecologic/oncologic surgeons will improve pretreatment assessment and posttreatment care in our elderly patients.

References

1. Jemal A, Murray T, Samuels A, Ghafoor A, Ward E, Thun MJ. Cancer statistics. CA Cancer J Clin. 2003;53:5–26.
2. Mcgonigle KF, Lagasse LD, Karlan BY. Ovarian, uterine, and cervical cancer in the elderly woman. Clin Geriatr Med. 1993;9:115–30.
3. Bristow RE, Tomacruz RS, Armstrong DK, Trimble EL, Montz FJ. Survival effect of maximal cytoreductive surgery for advanced ovarian carcinoma during the platinum era: a meta-analysis. J Clin Oncol. 2002;20:1248–59.
4. Chi DS, Eisenhauer EL, Zivanovic O, et al. Improved progression-free and overall survival in advanced ovarian cancer as a result of a change in surgical paradigm. Gynecol Oncol. 2009;114:26–31.
5. Ries LAG, Harkins D, Krapcho M, et al. SEER cancer statistics review, 1975–2003. Bethesda: National Cancer Institute; 2005.
6. Hightower RD, Nguyen HN, Averette HE, et al. National survey of ovarian carcinoma. IV: patterns of care and related survival for older patients. Cancer. 1994;73:377–83.
7. Thigpen T, Brady MF, Omura GA, et al. Age as a prognostic factor in ovarian carcinoma. The Gynecologic Oncology Group experience. Cancer. 1993;71:606–14.
8. Pignata S, Vermorken JB. Ovarian cancer in the elderly. Crit Rev Oncol Hematol. 2004;49:77–86.
9. Trillsch F, et al. Treatment reality in elderly patients with advanced ovarian cancer: a prospective analysis of the OVCAD consortium. J Ovarian Res. 2013;6:42.
10. Du Bois A, Reuss A, Pujade-Lauraine E, Harter P, Ray-Coquard I, Pfisterer J. Role of surgical outcome as prognostic factor in advanced epithelial ovarian cancer: a combined exploratory

analysis of 3 prospectively randomized phase 3 multicenter trials: by the Arbeitsgemeinschaft Gynaekologische Onkologie Studiengruppe Ovarialkarzinom (AGOOVAR) and the Groupe d'Investigateurs Nationaux Pour les Etudes des Cancers de l'Ovaire (GINECO). Cancer. 2009;115:1234–44.

11. Ries LAG, Reisner MP, Kosary CL, et al. Seer cancer statistics review, 1973–1999. Bethesda: National Cancer Institute. http://seer.cancer.gov/csr/1973_1999/2002. Accessed 15 Mar 2013.

12. Fried TR, Bradley EH, Towle VR, et al. Understanding the treatment preferences of seriously ill patients. N Engl J Med. 2002;346:1061–6.

13. Lichtman SM. Clinical trial design in older adults with cancer: the need for new paradigms. J Geriatr Oncol. 2012;3:368–75. 3,4.

14. Pallis AG, Fortpied C, Wedding U, van Nes MC, Penninckx B, Ring A, Lacombe D, Monfardini S, Scalliet P, Wildiers H. EORTC elderly task force position paper: approach to the older cancer patient. Eur J Cancer. 2010;46:1502–13.

15. Hutchins LF, Unger JM, Crowley JJ, et al. Underrepresentation of patients 65 years of age or older in cancer-treatment trials. N Engl J Med. 1999;341:2061–7.

16. Talarico L, Chen G, Pazdur R. Enrollment of elderly patients in clinical trials for cancer drug registration: a 7-year experience by the US Food and Drug Administration. J Clin Oncol. 2004;22:4626–31.

17. Siu LL, Tannock IF. Problems in interpreting clinical trials. In: Crowley J, editor. Handbook of statistics in clinical oncology. New York: Marcel Dekker Inc; 2001. p. 473–91.

18. Yee KWL, Pater JL, Pho L, et al. Enrollment of older patients in cancer treatment trials in Canada: why is age a barrier? J Clin Oncol. 2003;21(8):1618–23.

19. Wildiers H, Highley MS, de Bruijn EA, et al. Pharmacology of anticancer drugs in the elderly population. Clin Pharmacokinet. 2003;42(14):1213–42.

20. Brenner BM, Meyer TW, Hostetter TH. Dietary protein intake and the progressive nature of kidney disease: the role of hemodynamically mediated glomerular injury in the pathogenesis of progressive glomerular sclerosis in aging, renal ablation, and intrinsic renal disease. N Engl J Med. 1982;307(11):652–9.

21. Deppermann KM. Influence of age and comorbidities on the chemotherapeutic management of lung cancer. Lung Cancer. 2001;33 Suppl 1:S115–20.

22. Extermann M, Balducci L, Lyman GH. What threshold for adjuvant therapy in older breast cancer patients? J Clin Oncol. 2000;18(8):1709–17.

23. Piccirillo JF, Tierney RM, Costas I, et al. Prognostic importance of comorbidity in hospital-based cancer registry. JAMA. 2004;291(20):2441–7.

24. Kornblith AB, Kemeny M, Peterson BL, et al. Survey of Oncologists' perceptions of barriers to accrual of older patients with breast carcinoma to clinical trials. Cancer. 2002;95:989–96.

25. Lewis JH, Kilgore ML, Goldman DP, et al. Participation of patients 65 years of age or older in cancer clinical trials. J Clin Oncol. 2003;21:1383–9.

26. Makary MA, Segev DL, Pronovost PJ, et al. Frailty as a predictor of surgical outcomes in older patients. J Am Coll Surg. 2010;210:901–8.

27. Robinson TN, Eiseman B, Wallace JI, et al. Redefining geriatric preoperative assessment using frailty, disability and co-morbidity. Ann Surg. 2009;250:449–55.

28. Robinson TN, Wallace JI, Wu DS, et al. Accumulated frailty characteristics predict postoperative discharge institutionalization in the geriatric patient. J Am Coll Surg. 2011;213:37–44.

29. Balducci L. Geriatric Oncology: challenges for the new century. Eur J Cancer. 2000;36(14):1741–54.

30. Lipsitz LA. Physiological complexity, aging, and the path to frailty. Sci Aging Knowledge Environ. 2004;16:pe16.

31. Flood KL, Carroll MB, Le CV, et al. Polypharmacy in hospitalized older adult cancer patients: experience from a prospective, observational study of an oncology-acute care for elders unit. Am J Geriatr Pharmacother. 2009;7:151–8.

32. Carreca I, Balducci L, Extermann M. Cancer in the older person. Cancer Treat Rev. 2005;31(5):380–402.

33. Extermann M, Hurria A. Comprehensive geriatric assessment for older patients with cancer. J Clin Oncol. 2007;25(14):1824–31.
34. Brunello A, Sandri R, Extermann M. Multidimensional geriatric evaluation for older cancer patients as a clinical and research tool. Cancer Treat Rev. 2009;35:487–92.
35. Stuck AE, Siu AL, Wieland GD, et al. Comprehensive geriatric assessment: a meta-analysis of controlled trials. Lancet. 1993;342(8878):1032–6.
36. Extermann M, Meyer J, Mcginnis M, et al. A comprehensive geriatric intervention detects multiple problems in older breast cancer patients. Crit Rev Oncol Hematol. 2004;49:69–75.
37. Winkelmann N, Petersen I, Kiehntopf M, et al. Results of comprehensive geriatric assessment effect survival in patients with malignant lymphoma. J Cancer Res Clin Oncol. 2011;137:733–8.
38. Freyer G, Geay JF, Touzet S, et al. Comprehensive geriatric assessment predicts tolerance to chemotherapy and survival in elderly patients with advanced ovarian carcinoma: a GINECO study. Ann Oncol. 2005;16:1795–800.
39. Trédan O, Geay JF, Touzet S, et al. Carboplatin cyclophosphamide or carboplatin paclitaxel in elderly with advanced ovarian cancer? Analysis of two consecutive trials from the GINECO. Ann Oncol. 2007;18:256–62.
40. Versteeg KS, Konings IR, Lagaay AM, van de Loosdrecht AA, Verheul HMW. Prediction of treatment related toxicity and outcome with geriatric assessment in elderly patients with solid malignancies treated with chemotherapy: a systematic review. Annals of Oncology Advance Access published February 25. Ann Oncol. 2014;00:1–5.
41. Extermann M, Boler I, Reich RR, et al. Predicting the risk of chemotherapy toxicity in older patients: the chemotherapy risk assessment scale for high-age patients (CRASH) score. Cancer. 2012;118:3377–86.
42. Hurria A, Togawa K, Mohile SG, et al. Predicting chemotherapy toxicity in older adults with cancer: a prospective multicenter study. J Clin Oncol. 2011;29:3457–65.
43. Kohne CH, Folprecht G, Goldberg RM, et al. Chemotherapy in elderly patients with colorectal cancer. Oncologist. 2008;13(4):390–402.
44. Repetto L, Venturino A, Fratino L, et al. Geriatric oncology: a clinical approach to the older patient with cancer. Eur J Cancer. 2003;39(7):870–80.
45. Basso U, Falci C, Brunello A, et al. Prognostic value of multidimensional geriatric assessment (MGA) on survival of a prospective cohort of 880 elderly cancer patients (ECP). J Clin Oncol. 2011;29(Suppl):9065.
46. Audisio RA, Pope D, Ramesh HS, et al. Shall we operate? Preoperative assessment in elderly cancer patients (PACE) can help. A SIOG surgical task force prospective study. Crit Rev Oncol Hematol. 2008;65:156–63.
47. Pope D, Ramesh H, Gennari R, et al. Pre-operative assessment of cancer in the elderly (PACE): a comprehensive assessment of underlying characteristics of elderly cancer patients prior to elective surgery. Surg Oncol. 2006;15:189–97.
48. Tre'Dan O, Geay JF, Touzet S, et al. Carboplatin/cyclophosphamide or carboplatin/paclitaxel in elderly patients with advanced ovarian cancer? Analysis of two consecutive trials from the Groupe d'Investigateurs Nationaux pour l'Etude des Cancers Ovariens. Ann Oncol. 2007;18:256–62.
49. Falandry C, Weber B, Savoye A-M, Tinquaut F, Tredan O, Sevin E, Stefani L, Savinelli F, Atlassi M, Salvat J, Pujade-Lauraine E, Freyer G. Development of a geriatric vulnerability score in elderly patients with advanced ovarian cancer treated with first-line carboplatin: a GINECO prospective trial. Ann Oncol. 2013;00:1–6.
50. Saliba D, Elliott M, Rubenstein LZ, et al. The vulnerable elders survey: a tool for identifying vulnerable older people in the community. J Am Geriatr Soc. 2001;49(12):1691–9.
51. Slaets JP. Vulnerability in the elderly: frailty. Med Clin North Am. 2006;90(4):593–601.
52. Soubeyran P, Bellera CA, Gregoire F, et al. Validation of a screening test for elderly patients in oncology. J Clin Oncol. 2008;26:730s (Suppl. 20). abstr 20568).
53. Extermann M, Aapro M, Bernabei R, Cohen HJ, Droz JP, Lichtman S, et al. Use of compre- hensive geriatric assessment in older cancer patients: recommendations from the task force on

CGA of the International Society of Geriatric Oncology (SIOG). Crit Rev Oncol Hematol. 2005;55(3):241–52.

54. Martin JF, Henderson WG, Zacharski LR. Accrual of patients into a multihospital cancer clinical trial and its implications on planning future studies. Am J Clin Oncol. 1984;7:173–82.

55. Hughes KS, Schnaper LA, Berry D, Cirrincione C, Mccormick B, Shank B, et al. Lumpectomy plus tamoxifen with or without irradiation in women 70 years of age or older with early breast cancer. N Engl J Med. 2004;351(10):971–7.

56. Vose JM, Armitage JO, Weisenburger DD, Bierman PJ, Sorensen S, Hutchins M, et al. The importance of age in survival of patients treated with chemotherapy for aggressive non-Hodgkin's lymphoma. J Clin Oncol. 1988;6(12):1838–44.

57. Satariano WA, Ragland DA. The effect of comorbidity on 3-year survival of women with primary breast cancer. Ann Intern Med. 1994;120(2):104–10.

58. Burris III HA, Moore MJ, Andersen J, Green MR, Rothenberg ML, Modiano MR, et al. Improvements in survival and clinical benefit with gemcitabine as first-line therapy for patients with advanced pancreas cancer: a randomized trial. J Clin Oncol. 1997;15(6):2403–13.

59. Tannock IF, Osoba D, Stockler MR, Ernst DS, Neville AJ, Moore MJ, et al. Chemotherapy with mitoxantrone plus prednisone or prednisone alone for symptomatic hormone-resistant prostate cancer: a Canadian randomized trial with palliative end points. J Clin Oncol. 1996;14(6):1756–64.

60. Tannock IF, de Wit R, Berry WR, Horti J, Pluzanska A, Chi KN, et al. Docetaxel plus prednisone or mitoxantrone plus prednisone for advanced prostate cancer. N Engl J Med. 2004;351(15):1502–12.

61. Balducci L. Geriatric Oncology. Crit Rev Oncol Hematol. 2003;46:211–20.

62. Wheelwright S, Darlington AS, Fitzsimmons D, Fayers P, Arraras JI, Bonnetain F, Brain E, Bredart A, Chie WC, Giesinger J, Hammerlid E, O'Connor SJ, Oerlemans S, Pallis A, Reed M, Singhal N, Vassiliou V, Young T, Johnson C. Br J Cancer. 2013;109(4):852–8.

63. Roila F, Tonato M, Basurto C, et al. Anti-emetic activity of high-dose of metoclopramide combined with methylprednisolone versus metoclopramide alone in cisplatin-treated cancer patients. J Clin Oncol. 1987;5:141–9.

64. van der Hoop RG, van der Burg ME, ten Bokkel Hinink WW. Incidence of neuropathy in 395 patients with ovarian cancer treated with or without cisplatin. Cancer. 1990;66:1697–702.

65. Tuxen MK, Hansen SW. Complications of treatment: neurotoxicity secondary to antineoplastic drugs. Cancer Treat Rev. 1994;20:191–214.

66. Lichtman SM, Wildiers H, Launay-Vacher V, et al. International Society of Geriatric Oncology (SIOG) recommendations for the adjustment of dosing in elderly cancer patients with renal insufficiency. Eur J Cancer. 2007;43(1):14–34.

67. Grieshaber CK, Grever MR. Toxicology by organ system. In: Holland JF, Frei E, editors. Cancer medicine. 5th ed. Hamilton/New York: B.C. Decker; 2000.

68. Boparai M, Lichtman SM. Geriatric medication management: evaluation of pharmacist interventions and potentially inappropriate medication (PIM) use in older (≥65 years) cancer patients. J Clin Oncol. 2009;27:15s. Suppl.; abstr 9507.

69. Vestal RE. Aging and pharmacology. Cancer. 1997;80(7):1302–10.

70. Flockhart DA, Tanus-Santos JE. Implications of cytochrome P450 interactions when prescribing medication for hypertension. Arch Intern Med. 2002;162(4):405–12.

71. King RS. Drug interactions with cancer chemotherapy. Cancer Pract. 1995;3(1):57–9.

72. Kivisto KT, Kroemer HK, Eichelbaum M. The role of human cytochrome P450 enzymes in the metabolism of anticancer agents: implications for drug interactions. Br J Clin Pharmacol. 1995;40(6):523–30.

Biological Research: Current Directions

9

Claire Falandry, M. Bonnefoy, Gilles Freyer, and E. Gilson

Contents

C. Falandry, MD, PhD (✉) • M. Bonnefoy
Geriatrics Unit, CarMEN Laboratory, Lyon Sud University Hospital, Lyon University,
Pierre-Bénite, France
e-mail: claire.falandry@chu-lyon.fr

G. Freyer
HCL Cancer Institute, Medical Oncology, and Université de Lyon,
Lyon, France

E. Gilson
Institute for Research on Cancer and Aging Nice (IRCAN), Université de Nice-Sophia
Antipolis, UMR 7284 CNRS, U1081 INSERM, Nice, France

Department of Medical Genetics, Archet 2 Hospital, Centre Hospalier Universitaire de Nice,
Nice, France

© Springer International Publishing Switzerland 2016
G. Freyer (ed.), *Ovarian Cancer in Elderly Patients*,
DOI 10.1007/978-3-319-23588-2_9

Introduction

Ovarian cancer treatment has progressed considerably over the past 10 years. Substantial changes in treatment guidelines are attributable to the advent of targeted therapies. This revolution was accompanied by a serious effort to understand the biological drivers of tumour development and progression. Of these, senescence and ageing pathways are good candidates for exploration using age-related tumor models. In this respect, ovarian physiopathology affords a model system that may allow us to better understand senescence pathways and the impact thereof both loss of fecundity and cancer development. As ovarian cancer demographics peak at older ages, it is tempting to speculate that a relationship exists between senescence and cancer.

Cancer treatment in the elderly is always associated with the question of how to assess geriatric populations and how to use such assessments to plan treatment. Again, modern biology may provide objective tools facilitating such work: biomarkers of aging must be defined.

This review will seek to answer two principal questions:

- How do ovarian ageing and ovarian carcinogenesis illuminate the theories of ageing?
- Are biomarkers of aging clinically relevant in the context of ovarian cancer?

Ovarian Biology and the Theories of Ageing

Various theories on aging have been formulated, commencing in the early 1950s. Modern biology has provided some support for all theories; illustrative examples and proofs-of- concept have been described. In the field of ovarian biology, in particular, it is tempting to speculate that a relationship exists between senescence and cancer development. Ovarian cancers increase in number after menopause and peak at 70–80 years of age. From a biological viewpoint, menopause is a consequence of ovarian germ cell senescence, and a complex relationship is known to exist between senescence and cancer; senescence is both a barrier to cancer and tumor-promoting in nature. This section will describe the various theories of aging, again developed from the 1950s, and provide current illustrations thereof in the context of tumor biology and, in particular, ovarian cancer.

From Historical Theories of Aging to Modern Biology

Ovarian Ageing: Different Cell Lines - Different Points of View

Ovarian ageing has been extensively studied because of the triple impact on fertility, menopause, and associated cardiovascular risks, and ovarian cancer. Briefly, the ovary comprises various cellular components, including germ, granulosa, stromal, and ovarian surface epithelial (OSE) cells [1]. Premature ovarian failure (POF) is considered as a model of premature ageing and is caused by premature senescence of germ cells, induced by senescence signaling in a particular micro-environment (stromal cells). It is believed that exposure of oocytes to an aged ovarian microenvironment triggers a female age-dependent process termed "reproductive aging" or "maternal aging" [2]. OSE cells regulate the secretion and transport of 17β-hydroxysteroid dehydrogenase and were recently shown to be the major source of ovarian cancer; other cancers originate from fallopian tube epithelium [3] and granulosa cells [4].

The Mutation Accumulation Theory Supports Premature Ovarian Failure and Ovarian Cancer Pathogenesis

The *mutation accumulation* theory of Medawar, a Nobel laureate, maintains that aging is caused by accumulation of mutations, and that natural selection cannot eliminate mutations that exert no detrimental effects until late in life. This view was prominent in the 1950–60s, creating affiliated theories such as the *free radical theory* of Harmann and the *oxidative stress* theory. According to the latter theory, aging promotes cancer development, and mutations affecting aging may thus exert such effects.

Infertility and premature menopause induced by cytotoxic treatments in premenopausal women [5], by cigarette smoke exposure [6] and, (more generally) by oxidative stress [7], constitute models of accelerated ovarian ageing, and amply illustrate the mutation accumulation theory.

Oxidative stress triggered by ovulation induces repeated cycles of DNA damage in OSE cells [8] as do chemical agents such as methoxychlor [9]. Such stress is hypothesized to induce pre-malignancy. Thus, it is not surprising that inhibition of the DNA repair genes *BRCA1* and *BRCA2* (termed "BRCAness") via mutation, gene deletion, or gene silencing, affects cancer development. This is an illustration of the *mutation accumulation* theory in play. Mutations in tumor suppressor genes are not (or are poorly [10]) counter-selected because such mutations exert no detrimental effects on fertility.

The Antagonist Pleiotropy Theory

A theory developed by George C. William suggests that certain genes may be positively selected because they promote reproduction and genomic stability, but that such gene expression may be detrimental later in life. This theory is usually exemplified by the dual role played by $p16^{INK4A}$ or $p53$; the gene is responsible for genomic stability by triggering cell-cycle arrest during DNA repair and, eventually, apoptosis and senescence. However, such activities may cause tissue exhaustion and clonality restrictions later in life, promoting aging in tissues with high-level renewal turnover.

In the ovary, early senescence of stromal cells triggers germ cell senescence; this is a perfect illustration of antagonist pleiotropy. Early cessation of germline meiosis is indeed supposed to ensure the quality of the transmitted genome. Maintenance of high-level proofreading mechanisms in germ cell lines creates high risks of infertility and premature ovarian failure after exposure to high-level oxidative stress (please see below).

The Disposable Soma Theory

August Weissman was the first to conceptualize what was later described as the *disposable soma* theory by Thomas Kirkwood; this features the co-existence of different proofreading devices in somatic and germline cells. In the former cells, low-accuracy mechanisms allow energy saving, leading to accumulation of mutations and, eventually, cell deterioration or death, whereas high-quality proofreading is necessary in germ lines, to ensure maintenance of the species. Ovarian physiology fits well with such a *"wear and tear" theory of aging* because, in ovarian germline cells, early detection of a mutation triggers premature meiotic arrest and apoptosis. In line with this view, most ovarian cancers are derived from somatic cells and, in particular, OSE cells. Indeed, during fertile life, somatic OSE cells are subjected to constant high-level DNA damage [8].

One of the more prominent illustrations of the disposable theory is the discovery of the telomerase gene by E. Blackburn. Telomeres are complex nucleoprotein structures located at chromosomal extremities and dedicated to the protection thereof from the mutagenic risk associated with linear DNA (that may be recognized by the nuclear machinery as containing DNA breaks). Each round of chromosomal replication is associated with systematic telomere loss at the 5' extremity, leading to progressive telomeric attrition, which is compensated, to different extents depending on the cell type, by telomerase-dependant elongation of the truncated telomeres. In germline cells, telomerase is expressed at high levels, allowing long telomeres to be maintained in gametic cells. In somatic cells, however, low-level or no telomerase expression is associated with a high rate of telomere loss, triggering DNA damage that ultimately causes senescence or apoptosis. If this response fails, a second level of genomic protection is available for even shorter telomeres triggering cell crisis and death.

Mice programmed to synthesize abnormally short telomeres are compromised in terms of both fertility and embryonic development [11]. Moreover, the telomere reverse transcriptase is more highly expressed in oocytes from young females, and telomere length in oocytes declines with age [12, 13]. As the oocytes of adult females are believed to be principally post-mitotic, any significance of the observed reductions in telomerase expression and telomere length remains unclear. It is possible that increased oxidative stress during aging contributes to telomere shortening and dysfunction. Another outcome of reduced telomerase expression may be extra-telomeric in nature resulting in genome-wide transcriptional changes [14]. Therefore, it is important to better understand how the functions of oocyte telomeres are controlled. In this context, it is interesting that the death-associated protein DAXX, overexpressed in ovarian cancer cells, contributes to maintenance of genomic stability, prevention of cellular senescence, and ovarian oncogenesis, via an interaction with the Promyelocytic Leukemia Protein (PML) [15, 16]. As embryonic stem (ES) cells require DAXX and PML to ensure telomeric integrity [17], it may be speculated that these two proteins are also involved in telomeric maintenance in OSE cells, to protect such cells from senescence.

The Complex Relationship Between Senescence and Cancer

Senescence as an Anticancer Process

A protective role of senescence in the context of cancer is suggested by the fact that oncogene expression is sufficient to trigger senescence in primary human cells. The possible oncosuppressive effect of senescence is supported by a series of papers showing that pre-neoplastic lesions contain high levels of senescent cells [18–20]. Moreover, senescence may be a cytolytic process whereby cancer cells are eliminated by the immune system [21, 22]. From the perspective of ovarian cancer, recent data have confirmed that senescence protects against cancer because, as in most tumors, the senescence pathway is disabled in ovarian cancer cells, which are therefore immortal [23]. Recent data suggest that a synthetic progesterone receptor (PR) agonist exerts an oncostatic effect that depends on induction of senescence in such cells; the protein upregulates expression of p21 and the Forkhead-box transcription factor FOXO1 [23]. These data may explain how high levels of circulating progesterone and progestin-containing oral contraceptives protect against cancer. Moreover, PR and FOXO1 are frequently lost by ovarian cancer cells, further suggesting that these proteins play oncosuppressive roles.

Senescence Promotes Cancer by Cell-Autonomous and Cell-Nonautonomous Pathways

Apart from the oncosuppressive function of senescent cells, as illustrated by the high levels of such cells in precancerous tumors, increasing data support the notion that senescent cells *per se* exhibit a pro-oncogenic potential.

Cell-Autonomous Pathways
Upon long-term culture of human primary keratinocytes, Gosselin et al. found that post-senescent cells developed the capacity to develop spontaneous tumors; this was proposed to be a consequence of senescence-induced accumulation of reactive oxygen species (ROS) in cells refractory to apoptosis [24]. The idea that post-senescent cells might be cancer drivers has been extensively studied in mouse models and some

human tumors. The data show that senescence is prevalent in pre-malignant tumours, and that progression to malignancy requires evasion of senescence [25]. The issue of whether such intrinsic effects of senescent cells play roles during ovarian oncogenesis remains to be determined.

Cell-Non-autonomous Pathways

Upon cessation of proliferation, senescent cells display specific phenotypes including shape modifications and accumulation of β-galactosidase, which indicate that the protein synthesis patterns of such cells have been fundamentally modified. Increasing evidence links senescent cell-induced phenotypes with the autocrine and paracrine properties of such cells, involving the so-called SMS (senescent messaging secretome) or SASP (senescence-associated secretory phenotype). The latter phenotype, evident both *in vitro* and *in vivo*, has been shown to play dual roles in oncogenesis. On the one hand, the phenotype provokes development of a pro-inflammatory phenotype in neighboring immunological cells, which then exert anti-tumoral effects. On the other hand, the phenotype induces the epithelial-to-mesenchymal transition of, and invasion by, premalignant cells, and also proliferative or degenerative defects in non-senescent neighboring cells [26–31]. In terms of ovarian cancer, Ras-dependent secretion of the product of the chemokine growth-regulated oncogene 1 (Gro-1) by epithelial cancer cells is required for ovarian oncogenesis triggered by senescence induction in stromal fibroblasts [32].

The epithelial-to-mesenchymal transition has recently attracted increased interest in the context of ovarian physiopathology; Luo found that this transition played a role in enrichment of ovarian cancer stem-like cells [31]. However, it is not yet known whether the SMS and/or the SASP participate(s) in such a transition *in vivo*.

Renewing Ageing Theories: The Hyperfunction Theory of Ageing

According to the hyperfunction theory, age is associated with sustained stimulation of metabolic pathways (IGF1 mTOR), triggering development of phenotypes observed during aging (notably, cancer). Ovarian reproductive activity depends on metabolic pathway activities; caloric restriction promotes preservation of the follicle pool of adult female rats by inhibiting activation of signaling by the Mammalian Target of Rapamycin (mTOR) [33]. Notably, mTOR overexpression, and phosphorylation of the downstream target thereof, S6Kinase, have been demonstrated in both indolent and aggressive mouse tumors as well as human ovarian endometrioid adenocarcinomas, notably in the context of dysregulation of Wnt/beta-catenin and PTEN/PI3K signaling. In these models, tumor growth was significantly reduced by oral rapamycin treatment [34]. These data are in line with the ovarian findings; mTOR signaling plays a role in cancer development. mTOR inhibitors will be developed in future.

Are Ageing Biomarkers Clinically Relevant in the Context of Ovarian Cancer?

Ovarian cancer is a disease of the elderly; the incidence thereof peaks between the ages of 70 and 75 years. As aging is heterogeneous, being characterized by progressive declines in the functional reserves of many organ systems [35], surgeons and oncologists evaluate the reserves of each patient individually and adapt treatment plans accordingly. Comprehensive geriatric assessment seeks to monitor and correct geriatric vulnerability. Some authors propose that biomarkers of aging could be readily and reproducibly used to assess such vulnerability. Such biomarkers would be predictive of the loss of functional reserves, as revealed upon attainment of various endpoints including overall survival and/or functional disability.

Recently, two careful reviews on biomarkers of aging have appeared, although the interpretations differ somewhat [36, 37]. Briefly, aging biomarkers are usually markers of DNA damage and oxidative stress, telomere dysfunction, and senescence (particularly immunosenescence) and may reflect a genetic predisposition toward longevity. In the particular context of ovarian cancer, a French group investigating ovarian and breast cancer (GINECO) ran a prospective phase II trial evaluating the psychogeriatric vulnerability of elderly patients (over 70 years of age) on first-line carboplatin treatment for ovarian cancer; blood was systematically sampled for telomere length (TL) analysis. The working hypothesis was that TL could predict patient vulnerabilities and treatment outcomes. The exploratory study identified TL as predictive of decreased treatment completion, the risk of serious adverse events, unplanned hospital admission, and overall survival, after adjustment for FIGO stage (Falandry et al, in preparation). These results may perhaps be considered surprising, because TL was previously shown to correlate only weakly with survival in large longitudinal epidemiological studies. The significance of the association was both variable and demonstrable only when large numbers of patients were included. Thus, these results need to be confirmed in larger studies, and may lead to the construction of new hypotheses, perhaps proposing that tumors per se may accelerate organismal aging.

Conclusions and Perspectives

Recent advances in modern biology have shed new light on historical theories of aging. However, the light is both artificial and partial; no comprehensive view of ovarian aging and cancer development has emerged and new treatments thus remain elusive. Future work must explore aging pathways, disentangle the roles that they play in carcinogenesis, determine whether such pathways are relevant in real clinical situations, and gather epidemiological data. On another topic: biomarkers of aging would constitute a practical and relatively easy means by which biological age could be assessed at the level of the organism; the impact thereof on general patient outcomes could then be evaluated. Such markers would yield quantitative, reproducible, and rapid data guiding treatment decisions. However, few such data are presently available and our current challenge is to integrate ancillary translational studies into elder-specific trials.

References

1. Karve TM, Preet A, Sneed R, et al. BRCA1 regulates follistatin function in ovarian cancer and human ovarian surface epithelial cells. PLoS One. 2012;7:1.
2. Tatone C, Amicarelli F, Carbone MC, Monteleone P, Caserta D, Marci R, Artini PG, Piomboni P, Focarelli R. Cellular and molecular aspects of ovarian follicle ageing. Hum Reprod Update. 2008;14:131–42.
3. Przybycin CG, Kurman RJ, Ronnett BM, et al. Are all pelvic (nonuterine) serous carcinomas of tubal origin? Am J Surg Pathol. 2010;34:1407–16.
4. Chen VW, Ruiz B, Killeen JL, et al. Pathology and classification of ovarian tumors. Cancer. 2003;97:2631–42.
5. Letourneau J, Chan SW, Rosen MP. Accelerating ovarian age: cancer treatment in the premenopausal woman. Semin Reprod Med. 2013;31:462–8.
6. Sobinoff AP, Beckett EL, Jarnicki AG, et al. Scrambled and fried: cigarette smoke exposure causes antral follicle destruction and oocyte dysfunction through oxidative stress. Toxicol Appl Pharmacol. 2013;271:156–67.
7. Aiken CE, Tarry-Adkins JL, Ozanne SE. Suboptimal nutrition in utero causes DNA damage and accelerated aging of the female reproductive tract. FASEB J. 2013;27:3959–65.
8. Murdoch WJ. Carcinogenic potential of ovulatory genotoxicity. Biol Reprod. 2005;73(4):586–90.
9. Symonds DA, Merchenthaler I, Flaws JA. Methoxychlor and estradiol induce oxidative stress DNA damage in the mouse ovarian surface epithelium. Toxicol Sci. 2008;105(1):182–7.
10. Pavard S, Metcalf CJ. Negative selection on BRCA1 susceptibility alleles sheds light on the population genetics of late-onset diseases and aging theory. PLoS One. 2007;2:e1206.
11. Liu L, Blasco M, Trimarchi J, Keefe D. An essential role for functional telomeres in mouse germ cells during fertilization and early development. Dev Biol. 2002;249:74–84.
12. Hamatani T, Falco G, Carter MG, Akutsu H, Stagg CA, Sharov AA, Dudekula DB, VanBuren V, Ko MS. Age-associated alteration of gene expression patterns in mouse oocytes. Hum Mol Genet. 2004;13:2263–78.
13. Yamada-Fukunaga T, Yamada M, Hamatani T, Chikazawa N, Ogawa S, Akutsu H, Miura T, Miyado K, Tarín JJ, Kuji N, Umezawa A, Yoshimura Y. Age-associated telomere shortening in mouse oocytes. Reprod Biol Endocrinol. 2013;11:108.
14. Ye J, Renault VM, Jamet K, Gilson E. Transcriptional outcome of telomere signalling. Nat Rev Genet. 2014;15(7):491–503.
15. Pan WW, Yi FP, Cao LX, et al. DAXX silencing suppresses mouse ovarian surface epithelial cell growth by inducing senescence and DNA damage. Gene. 2013;526:287–94.
16. Pan WW, Zhou JJ, Liu XM, Xu Y, Guo LJ, Yu C, Shi QH, Fan HY. Death domain-associated protein DAXX promotes ovarian cancer development and chemoresistance. J Biol Chem. 2013;288(19):13620–30.
17. Ivanauskiene K, Delbarre E, McGhie JD, Küntziger T, Wong LH, Collas P. The PML-associated protein DEK regulates the balance of H3.3 loading on chromatin and is important for telomere integrity. Genome Res. 2014;24(10):1584–94.
18. Prieur A, Peeper DS. Cellular senescence in vivo: a barrier to tumorigenesis. Curr Opin Cell Biol. 2008;20:150–5. Epub 2008 Mar 18, 2008.
19. Collado M, Serrano M. Senescence in tumours: evidence from mice and humans. Nature. 2010;10:51–7.
20. Xue W, Zender L, Miething C, et al. Senescence and tumour clearance is triggered by p53 restoration in murine liver carcinomas. Nature. 2007;445:656–60. Epub 2007 Jan 24, 2007.

21. Kang TW, Yevsa T, Woller N, et al. Senescence surveillance of pre-malignant hepatocytes limits liver cancer development. Nature. 2011;479:547–51.
22. Collado M, Serrano M. Senescence in tumours: evidence from mice and humans. Nat Rev Cancer. 2010;10:51–7.
23. Diep CH, Charles NJ, Gilks CB, Kalloger SE, Argenta PA, Lange CA. Progesterone receptors induce FOXO1-dependent senescence in ovarian cancer cells. Cell Cycle. 2013;12(9):1433–49.
24. Coppe JP, Desprez PY, Krtolica A, et al. The senescence-associated secretory phenotype: the dark side of tumor suppression. Annu Rev Pathol. 2010;5:99–118.
25. Gosselin K, Martien S, Pourtier A, et al. Senescence-associated oxidative DNA damage promotes the generation of neoplastic cells. Cancer Res. 2009;69:7917–25.
26. Parrinello S, Coppe JP, Krtolica A, et al. Stromal-epithelial interactions in aging and cancer: senescent fibroblasts alter epithelial cell differentiation. J Cell Sci. 2005;118:485–96. Epub 2005 Jan 18, 2005.
27. Bavik C, Coleman I, Dean JP, et al. The gene expression program of prostate fibroblast senescence modulates neoplastic epithelial cell proliferation through paracrine mechanisms. Cancer Res. 2006;66:794–802.
28. Krtolica A, Parrinello S, Lockett S, et al. Senescent fibroblasts promote epithelial cell growth and tumorigenesis: a link between cancer and aging. Proc Natl Acad Sci U S A. 2001;98:12072–7. Epub 2001 Oct 2, 2001.
29. Liu D, Hornsby PJ. Senescent human fibroblasts increase the early growth of xenograft tumors via matrix metalloproteinase secretion. Cancer Res. 2007;67:3117–26.
30. Coppe JP, Patil CK, Rodier F, et al. Senescence-associated secretory phenotypes reveal cell-nonautonomous functions of oncogenic RAS and the p53 tumor suppressor. PLoS Biol. 2008;6:2853–68.
31. Luo X, Dong Z, Chen Y, et al. Enrichment of ovarian cancer stem-like cells is associated with epithelial to mesenchymal transition through an miRNA-activated AKT pathway. Cell Prolif. 2013;46:436–46.
32. Yang G, Rosen DG, Zhang Z, Bast RC Jr, Mills GB, Colacino JA, Mercado-Uribe I, Liu J. The chemokine growth-regulated oncogene 1 (Gro-1) links RAS signaling to the senescence of stromal fibroblasts and ovarian tumorigenesis. Proc Natl Acad Sci U S A. 2006;103(44):16472–7.
33. Li L, Fu YC, Xu JJ, et al. Caloric restriction promotes the reserve of follicle pool in adult female rats by inhibiting the activation of mammalian target of rapamycin signaling. Reprod Sci. 2015;22(1):60–7.
34. Tanwar PS, Zhang L, Kaneko-Tarui T, et al. Mammalian target of rapamycin is a therapeutic target for murine ovarian endometrioid adenocarcinomas with dysregulated Wnt/beta-catenin and PTEN. PLoS One. 2011;6:9.
35. Balducci L, Extermann M. Management of cancer in the older person: a practical approach. Oncologist. 2000;5:224–37.
36. Falandry C, Gilson E, Rudolph KL. Are aging biomarkers clinically relevant in oncogeriatrics? Crit Rev Oncol Hematol. 2013;85:257–65.
37. Pallis AG, Hatse S, Brouwers B, et al. Evaluating the physiological reserves of older patients with cancer: the value of potential biomarkers of aging? J Geriatr Oncol. 2013;5(2):204–18.